"*Back to Butter* takes us back to school on what we need to know to begin to restore the health of our families. With wisdom, compassion, and expertise, Molly and Sandy inspire us, helping us to navigate the changing landscape of food and health. Keep this book tucked away in your kitchen so you can turn to it, like a good friend, for insight, inspiration, and information."

—*Robyn O'Brien, author of* The Unhealthy Truth *and founder of the AllergyKids Foundation*

"This book is daring, inviting, and simply offered. Join Molly and Sandy as part of their family, and begin a mighty journey."

—*Arash Jacob, D.O., healer*

"Molly Chester and Sandy Schrecengost make eating logical and intuitive, empowering us to return to our roots. It's difficult to argue with the wisdom of nature and traditional whole foods. The knowledge contained in this book is life changing and may profoundly affect our health."

—*Maggie Ney, N.D., co-director of the Women's Clinic, Akasha Center for Integrative Medicine, CA*

"Molly and Sandy's recipes are among some of my very favorites. Not only do their recipes work, but they are filled with flavors your whole family will love. With food to nourish the mind, body, and soul, *Back to Butter* will become a treasured favorite."

—*Carrie Vitt, author of* Deliciously Organic *and founder of deliciouslyorganic.net*

"It used to be that every great cook knew the importance of using butter and other traditional ingredients. For nearly half a century, however, this was lost. *Back to Butter* is like a sigh of relief—an old friend has finally returned home."

—*Joette Calabrese, homeopath, public speaker, and author*

"In *Back to Butter*, authors Molly and Sandy deliver a candid and heartfelt approach to addressing some fundamental questions: What is real food and how should it be prepared? And what are the advantages of nourishing oneself in this manner? The recipes and advice are carefully thought out to reflect the wisdom of our ancestors, with the book's photography further accentuating these important words. This book is a labor of love, both in writing and in living a lifestyle."

—*Raymond Silkman, D.D.S.*

"If there's one thing I wish all my patients knew, it's that healthy eating is one of the most critical, basic things we can do to promote good health, offering both immediate and long-term health benefits. *Back to Butter* is a rich resource in this regard, packed with wonderful, mouthwatering recipes, beautiful photographs, and pure, unadulterated nourishment."

—*Greg Merti, M.D.*

"I've often wondered how we went so far astray with the simple act of feeding ourselves. Unearthing the path to finding our way back to simple nourishment is like hacking through a forest of odd diets, claims, and products. *Back to Butter* cuts through the clutter to present a road to sane eating rooted in traditional diets."

—*Evan Kleiman, chef, author, and radio host of L.A.'s* Good Food

"I love to cook. And I love fresh, natural ingredients—no processed foods on my table! Finally, a wonderful, beautiful cookbook that helps me put it all together."

—*Ruth Graham, Christian author and speaker*

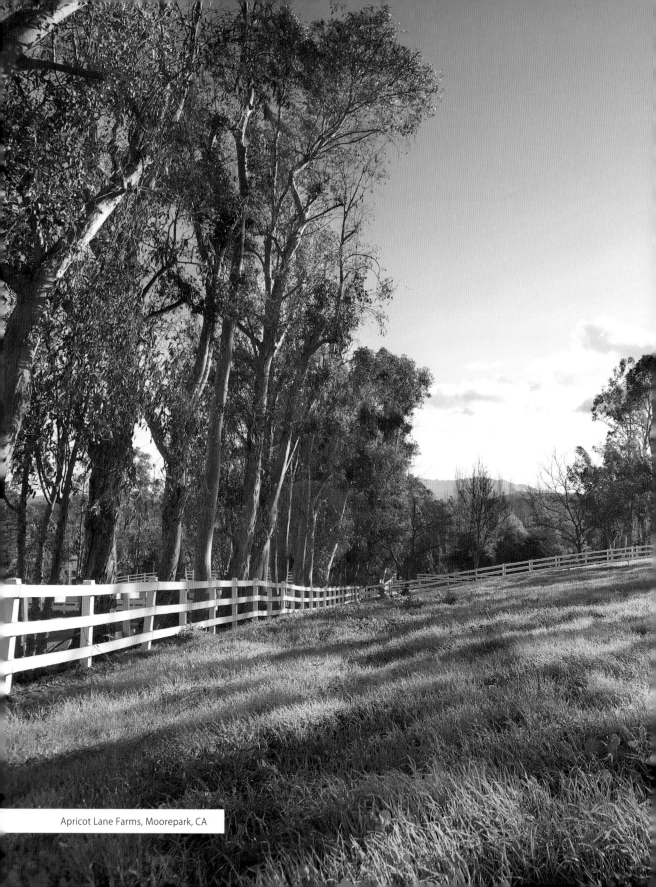

Apricot Lane Farms, Moorepark, CA

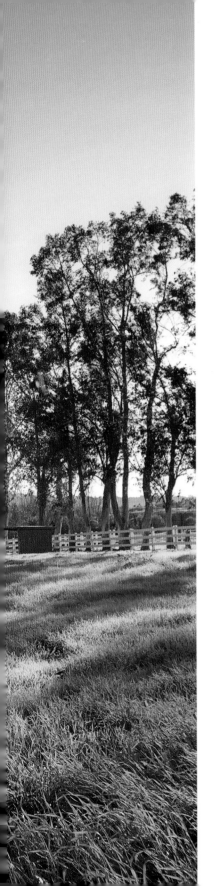

BACK TO BUTTER

A TRADITIONAL FOODS COOKBOOK
NOURISHING RECIPES INSPIRED BY OUR ANCESTORS

MOLLY CHESTER & SANDY SCHRECENGOST
FOREWORD BY BECK

Fair Winds Press
100 Cummings Center, Suite 406L
Beverly, MA 01915

fairwindspress.com • quarryspoon.com

First published in the USA in 2014 by
Fair Winds Press, a member of
Quayside Publishing Group
100 Cummings Center
Suite 406-L
Beverly, MA 01915-6101
www.fairwindspress.com
Visit www.QuarrySPOON.com and help us celebrate food and culture one spoonful at a time!

18 17 16 15 14   1 2 3 4 5

ISBN: 978-1-59233-587-9

Digital edition published in 2014
eISBN: 978-1-62788-013-8

Library of Congress Cataloging-in-Publication Data available

Cover and book design by Rita Sowins / Sowins Design
Photography by John Chester

Printed and bound in China

The information in this book is for educational purposes only. It is not intended to replace the advice of a physician or medical practitioner. Please see your health care provider before beginning any new health program.

For Earth and all her shepherds

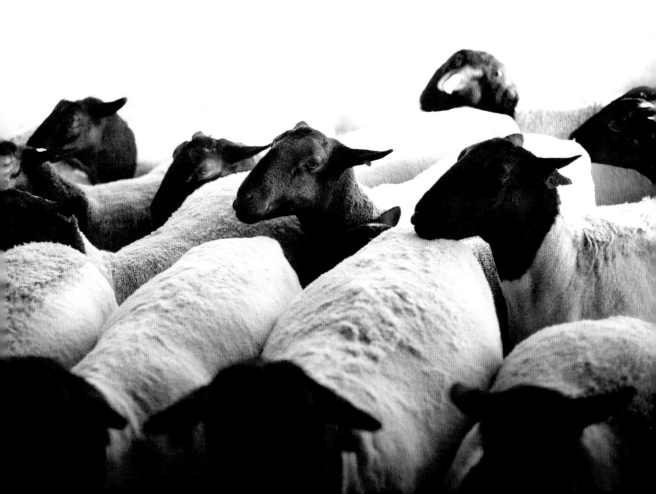

CONTENTS

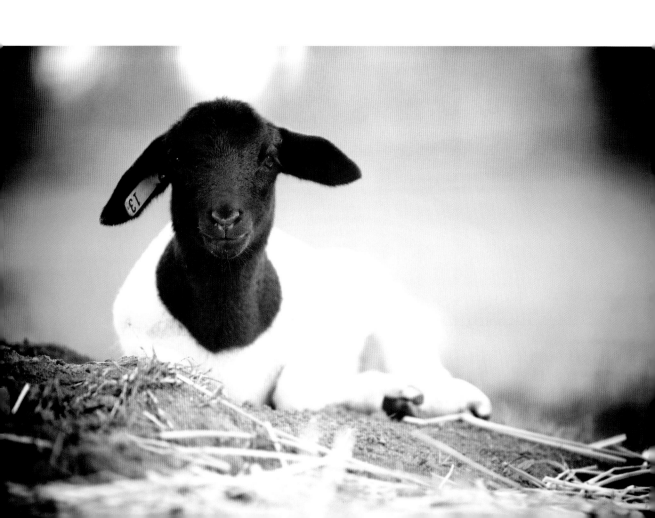

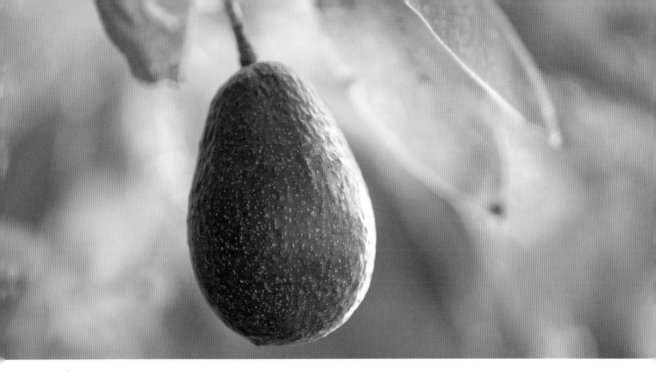

FOREWORD

Most people associate the name Beck with music, and not just any music, but trailblazing choices that carve new paths and remember classic beats. I do, too, but I also know my friend Beck, the one who understands food in a way that's reflective of the authenticity found in his art. I value his perspective and greatly appreciate his support of our work.

—Molly

From Beck:

A few years ago, Molly told me she was thinking about starting a farm. She had found a property outside of town and was considering taking on a new life. I wasn't surprised. It seemed like a natural progression from her work with food, a way of getting closer to the source.

Now she has written this book with Sandy, bringing together their experiences and what they've learned. Taking on a farm is tough work and the land has its own rules. These days, seeing the workings of nature firsthand is an experience afforded to very few. It's a perspective far removed from the shopper in the supermarket.

Food traditions are a reminder that there are always things to rediscover. In places like Spain or Japan, traditional foods are preserved and celebrated. You don't have to look hard to find people enjoying the same cuisine they've been eating for centuries. Traveling, it's apparent that the culture is in the food, the past is alive on the table. Molly and Sandy have been looking back at these traditions, and with this book, offer them back to us so we can appreciate them once again.

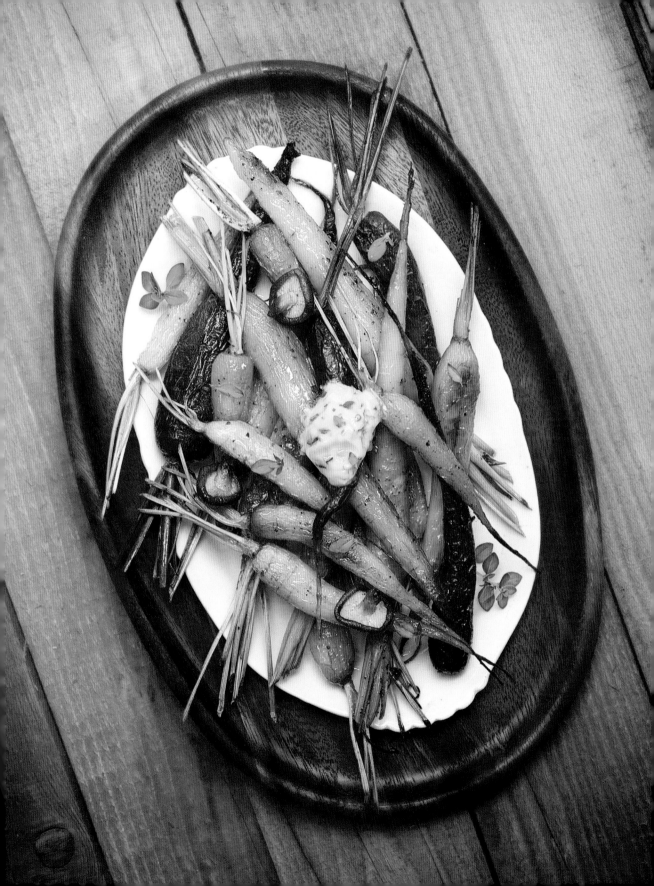

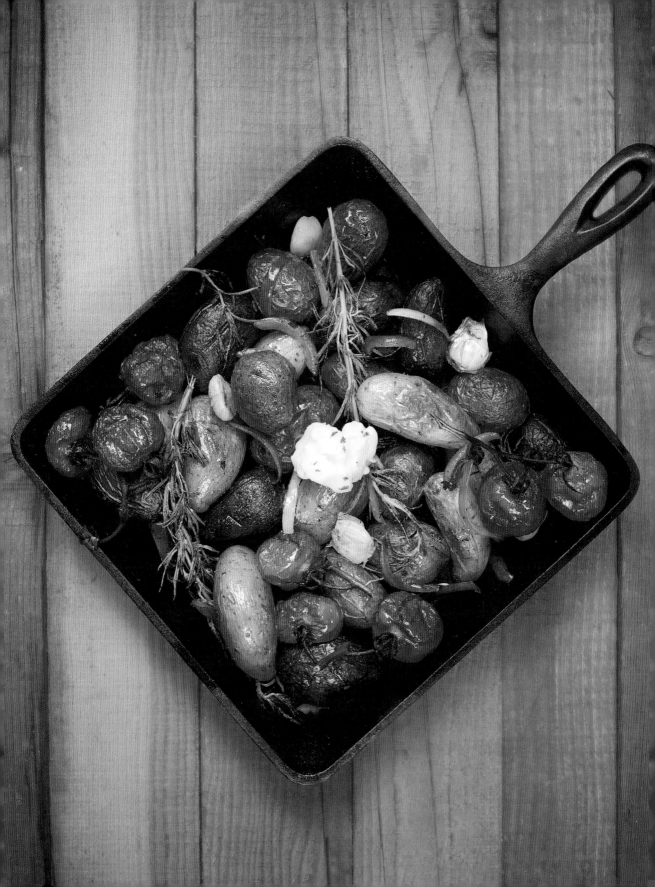

PREFACE

THE ONLY DIET THAT WORKED

It's not working, folks! We're feeling bad, and we're looking worse. Angry, diabetic, and depressed, we're disconnected from our food supply, and it's badly damaged our instincts. We're drowning in a sea of packaged products, antacids, and pain relievers, and something must be done.

The good news is there's a way out. It's a path that starts with taking responsibility for our own health, implementing sound, sensible nutrition into our lives, and (gasp!) returning to good ol' butter. My mom (and coauthor) and I have navigated our way back on track, and this book seeks to help you do the same.

I'm guessing that feeding your family is frustrating right now because it just doesn't make any sense. Simple things such as dairy, meat, and bread may be making you overweight, sick, depressed, and addicted. I (Molly) was there. I suffered under diagnoses such as polycystic ovarian syndrome (PCOS) and GERD (acid reflux), yet despite all efforts, my symptoms remained. I recall questioning, while in my mid-twenties, why I was so incredibly exhausted. Maybe you can relate. My life became increasingly rigid with vegetarianism, wheatgrass shots, and coffee enemas. Why was simple nourishment so unbearably complicated?

A few years later, while in culinary school, I purchased a book called *Nourishing Traditions* by Sally Fallon that pushed me toward an entirely different food paradigm. That book is a traditional foods encyclopedia of sorts, stressing the importance of nutrient-dense foods such as grass-fed meats, full-fat (raw) dairy, pastured eggs, and healthy fats. She shared "radical" ideas, including butter actually being incredibly good for you, and coconut oil and lard, too. These bastardized saturated fats were actually considered superfoods to our ancestors, as well as in long-lived traditional cultures around the world. Ms. Fallon's recipes, which included ingredients such as liver and chicken feet, defied yet intrigued my plant-based past.

Nourishing Traditions is inspired by the work of Dr. Weston A. Price, a prominent American dentist from the early 1900s who wondered why he was seeing so many dental problems in his patients—not only cavities and infection, but also what he called "dental deformities," that is, crowded and crooked teeth, overbites, and underbites. These findings, juxtaposed with the many reports he had heard of so-called "primitive people" from around the globe with beautiful straight white teeth inspired him and his wife to research the phenomenon.

Dr. Price located fourteen non-industrialized groups of people that had uniformly straight teeth, were free from cavities, and who exhibited excellent health overall. He then turned his attention to their diets. What kind of diet, he wanted to know, resulted in such obvious physical health?

His findings, documented in his book *Nutrition and Physical Degeneration*, revealed that while the diets of these healthy traditional peoples differed in the particulars—the diet of the Eskimos, for

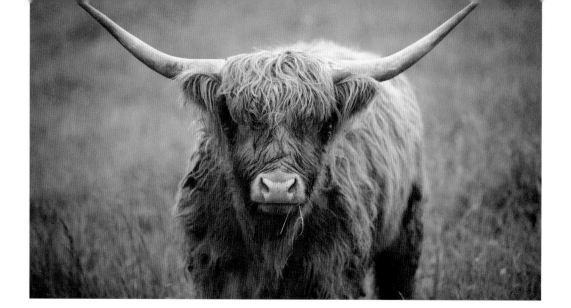

instance, relied heavily on fatty meats, organ meats, and fish, while those in the Swiss Alps ate more dairy and grains—the underlying principle remained the same: All the diets were extremely nutrient-dense, with particularly high levels of what he called the "fat-soluble activators," namely vitamins A, D, and K_2. Without these fat-soluble vitamins, the body cannot assimilate the minerals and water-soluble vitamins also in our food. Yet these fat-soluble vitamins are found in the very foods that we are often told *not* to eat: organ meats, butter, cream, egg yolks, fish eggs, animal fats, shellfish, and fish liver oils. Traditional peoples, on the other hand, held these foods to be sacred and particularly important for pregnant women and growing children.

When members of these "simple" societies left their native places and began eating processed foods, however, Dr. Price found that their health declined and cavities became rampant; children born in the next generation had more narrow faces and crowded teeth. Yet when people returned to their tribe or village and resumed their traditional diet, their health and vitality returned and their physical degeneration was reversed in the next generation. Holy smokes, right?

Dr. Price went on to implement some of the dietary practices he observed abroad in his own patients, using a combination of high-vitamin cod liver oil (rich in vitamins A and D) and an oil extracted from butter produced when cows grazed on lush spring grass (rich in vitamin K_2) to treat many diseases, including growth problems, infertility, arthritis, and seizures; he was even able to remineralize teeth and heal cavities with this combination.

When information makes logical sense, it becomes hard to ignore. Eager to find my own truth, I quit dabbling and became fully committed to this age-old food perspective, incorporating Dr. Price's principles—along with additional principles of healthy traditional diets described by other researchers and including things such as lacto-fermented foods, careful preparation of nuts and grains, use of gelatin-rich bone broths, and soulful farming and soil preservation—into my own meals. And I began, for the very first time, to feel stronger and infinitely more grounded. I literally stopped bumping into things. My energy leveled. And using personal trial and error, I eventually overcame each and every diagnostic

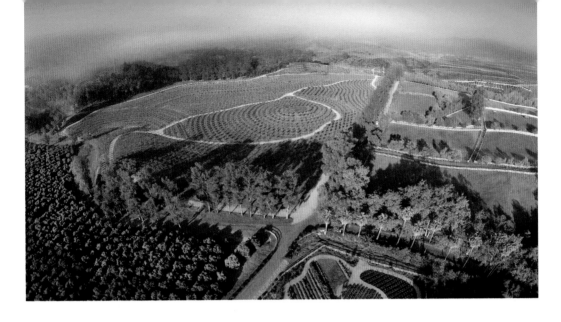

medical label. I humbly admit that we are each, forever, a work in progress, and many things take generations to unwind. But folks, my intense acid reflux and PCOS completely reversed. This was done without even one pill from conventional medicine, just food. Pretty powerful stuff.

Now, this next bit might seem a tad passionate because honestly, it was! In May of 2011, inspired by our "new" way of eating and our renewed appreciation for those who grow food, yet simultaneously puzzled by the limited availability of grass-based farmers, my husband, John, and I risked our established careers, moved to the country, and started to farm. It was the best decision we've ever made! Apricot Lane Farms (pictured above), a 160-acre (65 ha) gem in scenic Southern California, is farmed organically and biodynamically to produce extremely nutrient-dense and flavorful foods, pastured eggs, and more than seventy-five varieties of fruit trees. We'll be sharing tidbits from the farm throughout this book.

Prior to my farming days, I was a private chef for some of the biggest names in Hollywood (who, by the way, are beginning to embrace this information). I am not a scientist. Neither is my mother. She and I are simply cooks who have both overcome health issues by returning to Traditional Foods. Certainly, for every opinion, fact, and study, a counter-opinion, fact, and study can be referenced. But perhaps more importantly, what is the quality of the foods being used in these studies in the first place? Are grass-fed meats and pastured eggs, which could dramatically change the results of health studies, being sourced? Probably not. Therefore, while we wait for the smoke to clear, we simply request you open your hearts and ask yourself whether the information in these pages feels logical. And if so, does it make sense to you to give it a try? That's what we've always done.

The recipes in this book are favorites of our family and are filtered through the lens of the Traditional Foods movement. To ensure your success with these age-old techniques and ways of eating, Part I: The Traditional Foods Pantry (page 17) will carefully cover the basics. Overall, we encourage personal awareness and don't subscribe to the notion of a universal diet. Yet before you determine you cannot eat a certain food, I encourage you to read through everything and keep an open mind, because quality farming and the way that food is prepared can affect tastes and tolerances. Even a grain of wheat,

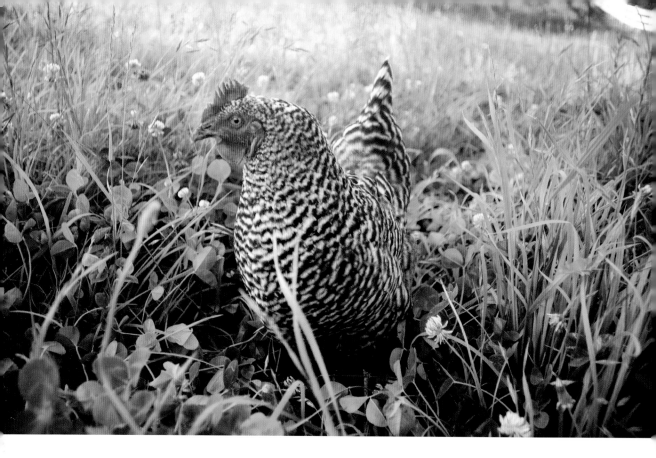

grown by a different farmer on different soil, can react differently to your body. It's quite possible, when eating the nutritionally rich version of a food that's been prepared traditionally, that your body may thrive.* What a gift would that be!

The Traditional Foods lifestyle flourishes when we surrender to the process. You will get no apology that many of these recipes take time. In fact, more time needs to be allocated to the important task of food preparation in the first place! The mind settles while soaking, rinsing, and spreading nuts onto dehydrator trays, or carefully culturing vegetables or dairy. A Nourishing Beef Stock (page 84) simmering happily on the stove offers contentment to anyone within sniffing range. Yet, in an effort to respect the balance of life, several of these recipes are family-friendly and downright speedy! Wisely approach your transition one step at a time, but remember this—somewhere in your historical genes, we believe you already know how to do this.

A bit of housekeeping to enhance your experience of this book: In order to avoid clutter, we decided to omit writing certain descriptive words into the ingredients lists of the recipes. For example, organic is not placed before, well, *everything*! But, we certainly recommend it be so. We recommend all meat and eggs be pastured, also known as grass-fed (page 35). All seafood is wild with sustainable certification, such as MSC (Marine Stewardship Council). All butter used in the creation of the recipes was pastured and unsalted. We highly recommend a quality mineral-rich sea salt, rather than refined

back to butter

14

> "Minerals in the soil control the metabolism of plants, animals, and man. All of life will be either healthy or unhealthy according to the fertility of the soil."
> —Alexus Carroll, 1912 Nobel Peace Prize winner

table salt. All vinegar is unfiltered and unpasteurized. All water is filtered. We recommend dairy be sourced as grass-fed, whole/full fat, and possibly raw, for uncooked applications (page 37). All flour, unless specifically noted, is soaked, sprouted, dehydrated, and then fresh-milled the day of use without ever being frozen. Lastly, we recommend raw honey (page 64) for all uncooked applications. When purchasing raw honey, we suggest sourcing a "pourable" type, which simply makes things easier. Many raw honeys are thick like peanut butter, which is delicious, but sometimes hard to stir into a recipe. Although many pourable honeys are not truly raw, there are definitely some that are both raw and pourable.

We feel grateful to have uncovered tools that heal our own bodies, and we're thrilled to share these seemingly magical tricks with you. Food holds the power to gradually change the trajectory of our future, and if we'd only listen, the proven successes of our ancestors can serve to inform our progress. Most of this groundbreaking information is not new to our world; we're simply starting to remember it.

Now, let's get cooking!

Although many of the principles of traditional foods are healing for the body, the mission of this particular book is to keep an already healthy body strong. For example, if you are looking to reverse PCOS, you may also need to cut out alcohol and sugar, even natural kinds, plus possibly lower your overall grain intake, or ramp up to quality fats more slowly, which is not reflected in this book. Find a good doctor who understands traditional foods, and then remember these foods were and are a critical element to our personal well-being, and they can be for you!

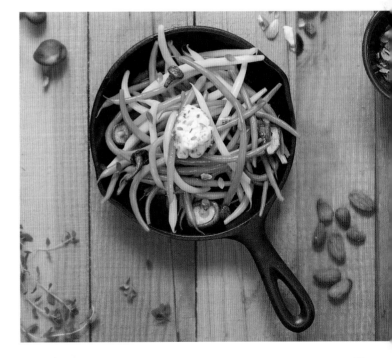

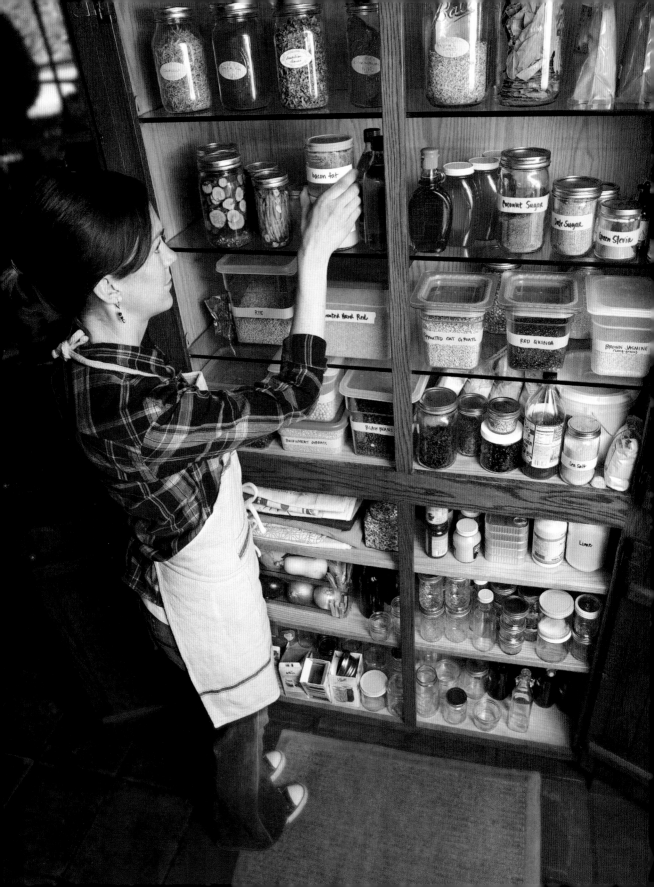

PART 1

THE TRADITIONAL FOODS PANTRY

What does *traditional foods* mean, you ask? The genre of traditional foods is powerfully emerging into the modern food landscape, yet the concepts on which it's based have strong, historical roots. Traditional foods utilize the culinary and farming techniques that consistently kept primitive cultures, cut off from the processed foods and medicine of modern societies, healthy, happy, and fertile. These techniques included grass-grazing animals; organic vegetable production; soaking grains, nuts, and seeds for improved digestion; drinking whole, raw dairy products; the inclusion of saturated fats and fermented foods; and more. These techniques may be new to you, and if a detailed explanation sounds helpful, know that's exactly what you'll find here. The Traditional Foods Pantry section of this cookbook is designed to thoroughly teach everything you need to know to master the recipes in part II. And while it helps to read over this chapter before you begin cooking, if you're more type B than A, we include page links within each recipe that connect back to each applicable technique, so either way, you're covered!

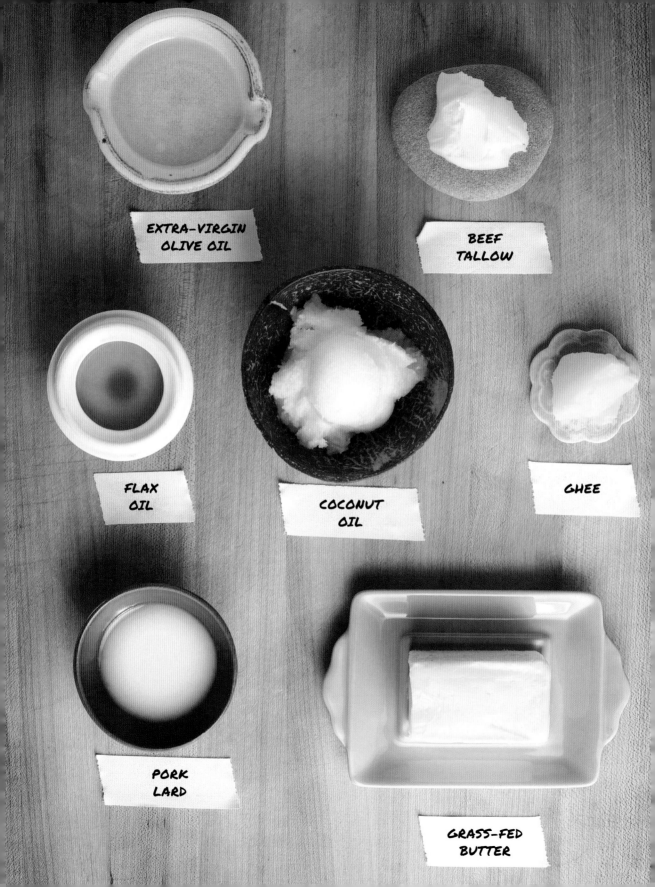

EXTRA-VIRGIN
OLIVE OIL

BEEF
TALLOW

FLAX
OIL

COCONUT
OIL

GHEE

PORK
LARD

GRASS-FED
BUTTER

CHAPTER 1

FATS & OILS

JOURNEY BACK TO UNREFINED FAT

On a very broad-stroke level, let's reflect back on our collective diets. One hundred years ago, the term *low-fat* didn't exist. The fats used in a typical American home were animal-based, namely lard, butter, and a bit of duck fat. Hold on to those thoughts while we digress …

Currently, two extremes seem to dominate our food culture. Let's give them team names. **Team Non-Fat Yogurt** debates every single calorie. Fat is the enemy, while weight and moods of their team members unpredictably waffle or stay steadily low due to an overall lack of consumption. This team is rightfully seeking health, but their definition of what creates it is distorting their results. On the flip side, **Team Fast Food** has never met a food label that couldn't be ignored. Though rightfully focused on simple enjoyment and good flavor, the offerings of our modern food supply hijack all health in the process. Dinner often prompts the question *where* to eat, instead of *what*. Team Fast Food's weight is inevitably very high, but surprisingly, a few malnourished skinny folks are on the roster as well. Regardless of how high or low the scale registers, however, the dismal reality is that both *Team Non-Fat Yogurt* and *Team Fast Food* are *undernourished* and ultimately, unsatisfied at the core.

To further our understanding of true nourishment, let's try an exercise. One afternoon, when the midday munchies attack, eat a juicy apple, a bunch of grapes, a few carrot sticks, and maybe a cucumber—as much as you want. Totally gorge yourself on fruits and vegetables. Afterward, monitor how long you remain satisfied. The next day at snack time, thinly slice one handful of radishes, top each with a sizable lump of grass-fed, full-fat butter, sprinkle on a little sea salt, and enjoy. Again, take note of how long you remain satisfied. *Spoiler alert:* the butter will likely win by a confident margin. This exercise reveals a very simple truth: fat makes us feel satisfied! And better still, despite what you may have heard, true, unadulterated fats don't actually make us fat—carbohydrates do.

Let's try another exercise. For two weeks, focus on raising the level of healthy fats in your diet, such as the ones we discuss in detail later in this section. Sauté all your vegetables in real butter, eat plain whole-milk, full-fat yogurt, and try bacon for breakfast with a side of eggs scrambled in the bacon drippings. *But avoid grains and sugar.* No bread. No dessert. No bagels. At the end of the week, check your belt notches. Feel a difference? You probably will. Now imagine doing the diet in reverse, forgetting about fat and instead focusing on raising the amount of grains and sugars in your diet. Doughnuts for breakfast, burritos for lunch, cake for dessert—you get the picture. Chances are, at the end of two weeks, you wouldn't need to check your belt because you'll already feel like a stuffed tick. Lesson learned: Healthy fats don't make us fat. Excess grains and sugars do.

But what about fried foods? If fats don't make us fat, why do we get fat when we eat too much fast food? Because . . . not all fats are created equal. Fats have something called a smoke point, which is a temperature at which the oil will literally smoke, burn, and turn rancid—and rancid oils are toxic to our bodies. Animal lard, for example, has a high smoke point, making it an ideal fat for the high temperature required for deep frying. Up until the late 1980s, a typical burger joint fried their onion rings and fries in beef lard (tallow). Nowadays, however, refined vegetable oil is used. The key word here is *refined*. Vegetable oils have a low smoke point, making them a terrible choice for frying. Therefore, low-smoke-point oils such as corn oil must be refined (*processed*) in order to handle that excess heat. But why go through all that trouble when tallow works perfectly fine without alteration? Because refined vegetable oils are dirt cheap, and therein lies the problem.

The substitution of refined vegetable oils doesn't seem to be making our society any healthier. As you can see, the goal of *Team Non-Fat Yogurt* might be health, but completely removing all fat (*and flavor*) from the diet isn't the answer. And while the goal of *Team Fast Food* might be flavor, we believe flavor can be achieved without sacrificing health.

Fat isn't to be feared. Fat is to be understood. Responsibility rests on the shoulders of each of us not only to step into the kitchen but also to form a basic understanding of real food, including fats. Because much of this information has been cast aside over the past several generations, let's examine each of the healthy, unrefined fats used in the Traditional Foods diet (and this cookbook) more closely.

FATS: THE BIG PICTURE

We must first gain a big-picture understanding of fats so that we can learn to properly use them in the kitchen. Two main categories of fats exist: saturated and unsaturated. To understand the difference between these two, think of a sponge. If water were slowly poured into a sponge until it couldn't possibly bear another drop, the sponge would be saturated. In the case of saturated *fat*, the fat molecule is the sponge, and it is filled up with hydrogen instead of water. Why does it matter whether a fat molecule is saturated with hydrogen? Because that's what makes it stable! In other words, saturated fat is like a party where everyone shows up with a date. No one is playing the field, and the party stays pretty tame. Unsaturated fat, on the other hand, is like a party where a couple of extra guys, a.k.a. dried-up sponges/molecules desperate for a bit of hydrogen, arrive solo. Unfortunately, now the numbers are no longer even—too many sponges and too little hydrogen. And when things heat up (literally) and there's not enough hydrogen to go around, this party's gonna get messy!

The stability or instability of the molecular structure of these two types of fats is in fact altered when temperatures rise. Stable saturated fats remain undisturbed by high heat, while the unstable molecular structure of unsaturated fat causes it to burn and break down quickly under relatively moderate temperatures. And as we've learned, burnt oil is rancid and unsafe for consumption. Although refinement can make rancid oil *palatable*, no amount of refinement can make it wholesome to consume. As such, unadulterated saturated fats are best for cooking, while unsaturated fats are best for low- to no-heat applications (such as salad dressings). Every fat has its place. We just need to know how to use them properly!

To complicate things a little bit, we must mention that fats and oils all contain *both* saturated and unsaturated fats in their constitution. Similar to how all human beings have both masculine and feminine properties, each fat is a mixture—yet they take on the characteristics of the dominant percentage. An easy way to determine whether a fat is more saturated or unsaturated is by analyzing its texture when at room temperature. Saturated fat is thick at room temperature, such as represented in lard, tallow, coconut oil, butter, and ghee. All of these fats contain a higher percentage of saturated fat. Unsaturated fat, on the other hand, is liquid at room temperature, as in walnut oil, sesame oil, flax oil, and olive oil.

Unsaturated fats also break down further into subcategories (polyunsaturated and monounsaturated), which affect each oil's composition, but in more subtle ways that are beyond the scope of this book.

UNDERSTANDING SATURATED AND UNSATURATED FATS

Saturated Fat = Stable = Thick at Room Temperature

Unsaturated Fat = Unstable = Liquid at Room Temperature

SMOKE POINT

The *smoke point* is the temperature at which a fat literally begins to smoke, burn, and turn rancid. Remember, rancid oils are toxic to our bodies. Although saturated fats as a whole have a higher smoke point than do unsaturated fats, individual fats within each category have their own unique smoke point, due to their specific ratio of saturated to unsaturated fat, as described above. For example, not all saturated fats are suitable for high-heat frying, and several unsaturated fats can handle the gentle simmer of a low flame. Below is a handy temperature legend for the fats used in this book, which we encourage you to apply to all cooking, not just the recipes here.

FATS TEMPERATURE LEGEND

Best for High Heat (e.g., frying onion rings): Ghee, Lard, Tallow

Best for Medium Heat (e.g., browning onions): Butter, Coconut Oil

Best for Low Heat (e.g., sweating onions): Extra-Virgin Olive Oil

Cold Use Only (e.g. raw onions): Walnut Oil, Sesame Oil, Flax Oil

A BREAKDOWN OF TRADITIONAL FATS

Several of the fats listed below, such as lard and tallow, are not as readily available as they once were. Though this is changing; please see Resources (page 216) for purchasing suggestions. Several mail-order options are quite reasonable and convenient, when local sources don't yet serve a community's needs. It won't be long until this concern is a thing of the past!

BUTTER: THE FRIENDLY FAT

TYPE: Saturated/Solid at Room Temperature

SMOKE POINT: Medium Heat

LOOK FOR: Organic, Unsalted, and Pastured/Grass-Fed

DESCRIPTION: Butter is a saturated fat that never should have fallen from grace. Its plastic counterpart, better known as margarine, entered our kitchens after World War II, and though it maintains its space on supermarket shelves, it is simply not real food. That said, not all real butter is created equal. The vitamin and nutritional content of butter made from the milk of cows that grazed on pasture under the open sun is far superior to that in the butter of factory-farmed cows. Instead of allocating funds for vitamins, consider purchasing a quality grass-fed butter, commonly known as pastured butter in the store. And when you find it, try the Fresh Herb–Crusted Sea Bass with Sourdough Bread Crumbs (page 118). Oh my!

CULINARY SYNONYM

To avoid confusion, we want to reiterate that *grass-fed* and *pastured* mean the exact same thing! It's sort of like 8 ounces (225 g) is just another way of saying 1 cup (225 g). So if you see one label or the other, you're good to go!

GHEE: BUTTER'S KIN

TYPE: Saturated/Solid at Room Temperature

SMOKE POINT: High Heat

LOOK FOR: Organic and Pastured/Grass-Fed

DESCRIPTION: When butter is gently simmered over low heat, the milk solids eventually fall to the bottom, leaving behind a clear yellow, clarified liquid called ghee. Because the milk solids have been removed, ghee has a higher smoke point than butter does and can be used to properly fry foods. The absence of milk solids also means that many lactose-intolerant people can tolerate ghee. As with butter, we prefer to use ghee made from the butter of grass-fed cows. Scallops brown beautifully with ghee, as in the Seared Scallops with Creamy Carrot Purée (page 114).

"The absence of milk solids also means that many lactose-intolerant people can tolerate ghee."

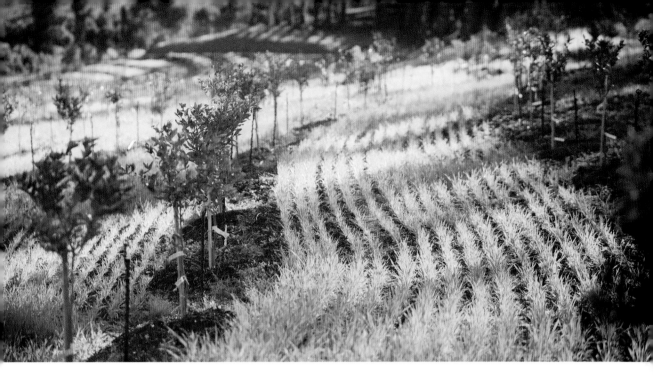

COCONUT OIL: A TROPICAL TREAT

TYPE: Saturated/Solid at Room Temperature

SMOKE POINT: Medium Heat

LOOK FOR: Organic, Unrefined, Virgin, and Centrifuged or Cold-Pressed

DESCRIPTION: Coconut oil contains both antifungal and antimicrobial properties that assist in keeping a family strong and resilient. The oil does have a mild coconut flavor, which can be masked when sautéing by folding in a bit of butter to the dish once removed from the heat. Conversely, its coconut flavor can also help a dish reach new heights, as in the Sprouted Apple Butter Dots (page 199).

PORK LARD: GRANDMA'S SUPERFOOD

TYPE: Saturated/Solid at Room Temperature

SMOKE POINT: High Heat

LOOK FOR: Organic and Pastured/Grass-Fed

DESCRIPTION: Pork lard is rendered and clarified pork fat. Not too long ago, pork lard was considered the key to the tastiest piecrust in town! And for good reason: Fats such as lard buffer the roller-coaster effect that carbohydrates and sugar have on the body, making them a wise choice for baked goods. As with purchasing pork (page 31), we prefer our pork lard to come from animals raised on pasture without the use of hormones and antibiotics. A simple recipe for collecting bacon fat, which is a seasoned version of pork lard, can be found on (page 33). In grandma's day, bacon drippings were typically saved and strained in order to fry the next day's eggs, or to build the crust of Sunday's quiche, or to sauté the dinner vegetables, which is the technique we use in our Brussels Sprouts with Onions and Crispy Bacon (page 166).

fats & oils

23

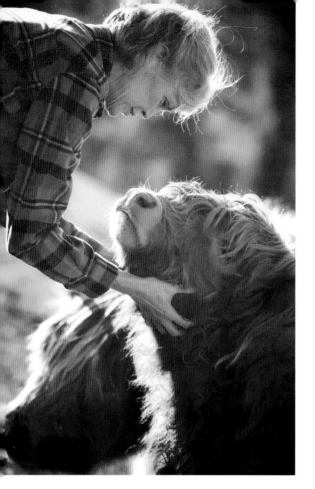

BEEF LARD, a.k.a. TALLOW:
THE UNREFINED FRYING OIL

TYPE: Saturated/Solid at Room Temperature

SMOKE POINT: High Heat

LOOK FOR: Organic and Pastured/Grass-fed

DESCRIPTION: Beef lard, also known as tallow, is rendered and clarified beef fat. Tallow has properties most closely related to those of pork lard and serves as an excellent substitute for people who choose not to eat pork products. As with purchasing beef (page 27), we prefer our tallow to come from an animal raised on pasture without the use of hormones and antibiotics. Beef lard fries food beautifully.

> "Don't be fooled by television chefs who use olive oil at high temperatures! The oil is either refined, or it is being used improperly."

EXTRA-VIRGIN OLIVE OIL: EVOO

TYPE: Unsaturated/Liquid at Room Temperature

SMOKE POINT: Medium Heat

LOOK FOR: Organic, Unrefined, Unfiltered, Virgin, and Cold-Pressed

DESCRIPTION: Extra-virgin olive oil is one of the more stable unsaturated fats, which remains liquid at room temperature but seizes up a bit when refrigerated. The important prefix *extra-virgin* implies that the oil is derived from the first pressing of the olives, resulting in the most nutritious oil with a lovely, delicate flavor. Don't be fooled by television chefs who use olive oil at high temperatures! The oil is either refined, or it is being used improperly. Get into the habit of using unrefined extra-virgin olive oil without heating by trying our Tangy Jam Dressing (page 112).

WALNUT OIL: A LIGHT AND LOVELY SEASONING

TYPE: Unsaturated/Liquid at Room Temperature

SMOKE POINT: Cold Use Only

LOOK FOR: Organic, Unrefined, Unfiltered, Virgin, and Cold-Pressed

DESCRIPTION: Treat yourself to a quality jar of walnut oil! We've found a small, local walnut farm that produces a beautiful variety (page 216), but any unrefined walnut oil will add light and lovely dimensions to a dish. Due to its delicate nature, walnut oil should be kept refrigerated. We use it primarily as a seasoning oil to enhance cold dishes, such as our Confetti Slaw (page 149), but it's also delicious when drizzled over a warm plated dish for a finishing touch.

SESAME OIL: A NUTTY AND FULL FINISHING OIL

TYPE: Unsaturated/Liquid at Room Temperature

SMOKE POINT: Cold Use Only

LOOK FOR: Organic, Unrefined, Unfiltered, Virgin, and Cold-Pressed

DESCRIPTION: As with walnut oil, use sesame oil as a salad or finishing oil. It imparts an intensely nutty flavor to a dish and is delicious drizzled over Traditional Hummus (page 74) or when complemented by Asian flavors, as in our Chilled Sweet 'n Sour Asparagus (page 150).

FLAX OIL: THE GOLDEN CHILD

TYPE: Unsaturated/Liquid at Room Temperature

SMOKE POINT: Cold Use Only

LOOK FOR: Organic, Unrefined, Unfiltered, Virgin, and Cold-Pressed

DESCRIPTION: Flax oil is a nutty oil with a slight bitterness that some may find unpleasant. But for those who enjoy the full-bodied flavor, it contains a generous amount of the nutritionally important essential omega-3 fatty acids. Use flax oil in healthy moderation with a variety of other oils. When shopping for flax oil, make sure the store keeps its bottles in refrigeration and note the sell-by date, because flax oil turns rancid easily, making the oil even more bitter and virtually unpalatable. It's best to buy small bottles of flax oil more frequently to avoid the waste of expiration. Flax oil is featured in our Raw Chopped Salad (page 104).

EMBRACE NEW FATS!

If you're anything like I was, the only fat on the above list that currently lives in your kitchen is extra-virgin olive oil. If that is the case, try purchasing one new fat with each trip to the grocery store. And if we've convinced you to put butter on your grocery list for the very first time, you're in for a real treat!

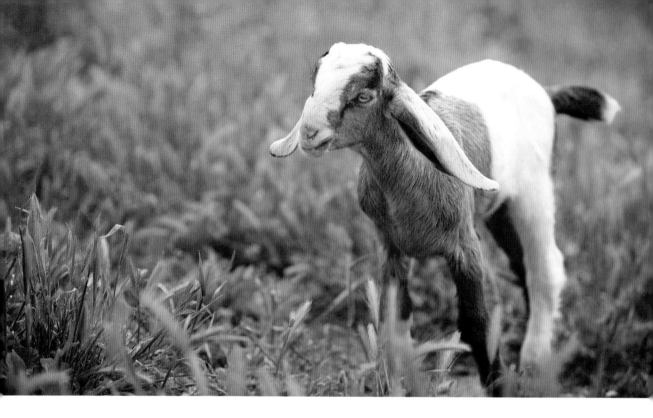

CHAPTER 2

SUSTAINABLE MEAT

HEALTHY ANIMAL = HEALTHY YOU!

John and I have a little black dog named Todd. Every day, sometimes all day, Todd saunters out to a sunny section of our courtyard, plops down, and takes in a big old dose of sunshine. When he's had his fill, he meanders over under the bougainvillea for a much-needed nap in the shade. This happens every single day. Todd needs his sun. Sheep, on the other hand, who are in the sun all day, really appreciate access to shade. They'll even create their own, when necessary, by standing in a huddle with their heads underneath their neighbor's stomach. Sheep are also extremely unhappy in a pasture that doesn't have a lot of quality grass. Without a bit of patience, they baa-aaa like an orchestra and stomp their feet while

back to butter

26

standing near the gate. And then there are the chickens, who tuck themselves in at night! Every evening at dusk, they go back to their mobile housing unit for shelter, completely unprompted—we simply close the door. But you better believe they are crowing and clucking loudly in the morning if we're even a few minutes late to open it back up. As for the cows, if they're in the pasture with green grass and a pile of dried alfalfa, they ignore the alfalfa and chomp on the fresh grass. Suffice it to say, they've all got opinions!

Just like us, animals need space, sun, shade, clean water, and appropriate food. Their behavior is almost always reflective of their attempt to solve one of those basic needs. When they can't remedy their own issues and no one does it for them, they begin to get sick, and when they get sick, they often receive antibiotics. But the question is, why do we turn so quickly to antibiotics before we've revisited the basics of quality space, sun, water, and food?

Animals who are compassionately raised have muscles and bones that are strong from proper exercise. And just like us, cows fed a proper diet don't feel bloated and gassy. When chickens forage pastures to eat bugs, clover and grass, the yolks of their eggs turn a magnificent bright orange, whereas factory-farmed yolks are a pale, pastel yellow. The yolk doesn't lie! And who benefits from this health? We do! We eat the animal. On a very basic level, the quality of the animal literally becomes the quality of us. We truly are what we eat.

With that said, attaining high-quality space, sun, water, and food for animals can be expensive, pushing the cost of quality meat higher. Personally, I budget high food costs as a necessity. "Food Costs" might as well merge with the "Medical" line item in my budget, under preventive care. Yet, sometimes, even necessities get cut. During those tight times, even one step in the right direction helps. We want to help you make that first step. Below are the categories of meat we use for the recipes in this book. Directly below each type of meat is a listing of the buzzwords we care about and look for when purchasing, and below that is an explanation of how we make our selections in each category. If all the buzzwords can be found pertaining to one farmer's meat, hooray! But if not, try adopting one at a time. Step into it, and soon, you may understand why we suggest seeking out a compassionate, thoughtful farmer and paying a premium for sustainable meats. It costs more because it's *worth* more.

BEEF

LOOK FOR: Local, Grass-Fed or Grass-Finished, and Organic

Cows, by nature, eat fresh grass. The cattle supplying most common grocery store beef, however, have been penned into small areas and fed grain, which is only the dried seed of grass, and legumes such as soy. Because mass amounts of grain and soy are not the natural feed for cows, and because their personal space is wholly disregarded, health and digestive issues ensue, prompting the need for antibiotics.

This vicious cycle feels unnatural, no? That's why we recommend avoiding it completely by purchasing meats from a farmer at a local market, whose eyes you can look into as you shake hands and ask if their cows graze on pasture (*meaning grass*).

When purchasing beef, look out for the term *grass-finished*, meaning that a cow has grazed on grass year-round with no grain supplementation. Grass-finished is top-notch, but grass-fed—wherein a cow's diet is supplemented with grain during the barren winter months—is still very high quality and slightly more realistic in some climates, and it doesn't seem to affect the cow's overall health. When we supplement with grocery store beef, we choose **local** (to avoid purchasing meat that must be shipped across the country), **grass-fed** (to ensure the cow received time on pasture eating grass) or even better **grass-finished** (in support of the cow receiving year-round pasture and grass), and **organic** (to avoid growth hormones and antibiotics).

EGGS

LOOK FOR: Local, Pastured, Organic, and Soy-Free

Back in the day, chickens frolicked the farm foraging for bugs and snails, eating a bit of grass, and maybe getting frisky with a rooster from time to time. That's natural and just makes sense. The term *pastured* defines the above description, but 100 percent pastured chicken eggs, unfortunately, are the hardest eggs to source. As always, my first suggestion is to visit a local farmers' market in search of 100 percent pastured eggs. If unavailable, try asking a friendly face at a local health food store for a listing of trusted local farms, or even hop on the Internet to do a search for pastured eggs in your area.

We recommend eggs as the very first food to source directly from a farm. The quality between eggs from chickens that are pastured versus grocery store eggs is so vastly superior that the effort completely pays off. The nutrition of a single pastured egg offers significantly higher levels of vitamins A, D, and E, as well as higher amounts of omega-3s, an element in which most diets are woefully deficient. This critical, essential fatty acid is a regulator of metabolism and a building block of the body that it cannot manufacture on its own.

When a chicken's diet relies on wild foraging, the yolks are almost orange. No lie. Once you see and taste the difference, it is very hard to go back! Keep in mind that it is expensive for a farmer to produce truly pastured eggs, which is why they cost more. Speaking from experience, I can tell you that the farmers are not making a killing off their eggs. Mobile coops, (one of ours is pictured on page 29), must be moved every few days, and the chickens must not be overcrowded. It is a labor of love.

When a local farm is unavailable, here are some words to look for on grocery store labels: **local** (to avoid purchasing eggs that must be shipped across the country), **pastured** (to ensure the chicken roamed the farm as chickens should) or at least **free-range** (to ensure the chicken received time, however limited, in sunlight), and **organic** (to avoid hormones and antibiotics). It's also preferred that the chickens not be fed soy, so look for the **soy-free** label as well.

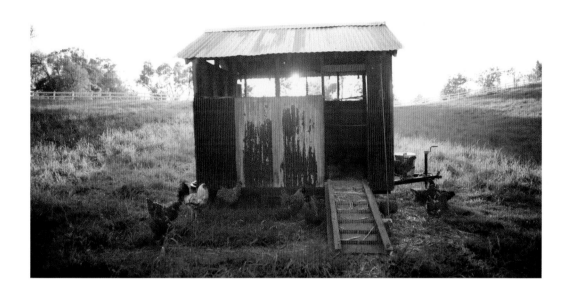

POULTRY

LOOK FOR: Local, Pastured, Organic, and Soy-Free

"We recommend eggs as
the very first food to source
directly from a farm. The
quality between eggs from
chickens that are pastured
versus grocery store eggs is
so vastly superior that the
effort completely pays off."

Broiler chickens, or chickens used for their meat, are raised slightly differently than layer hens, chickens used for their eggs, and here's why: Although 100 percent pastured chickens are the healthiest chickens in terms of exercise, they also don't have much meat on their bones for roasting because they've been running around so much! It *is* possible to find 100 percent pastured broiler chickens from a local farmer or even some health food stores, and I absolutely recommend using them for our homemade chicken stock (page 82), but for a delicious chicken that still receives moderate exercise, fresh green grass, and fresh air, I suggest finding a farmer who raises broilers in mobile pens, which are small bottomless coops that get moved to fresh green grass daily, but keep the chickens more contained. Although still technically referred to as **pastured** (how's that for confusion?), they result in a healthy, meatier bird that we feel represents a reasonable compromise.

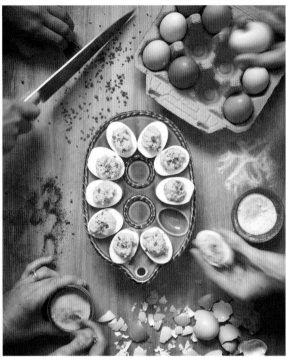
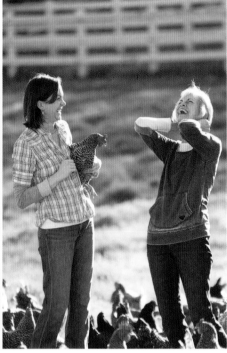

Most all chickens are fed supplemental grain, especially in the winter when the bug activity is down, but I personally prefer that the feed is **soy-free** (page 50). A few other poultry buzzwords commonly used in grocery stores are **cage-free**, which is not regulated and really doesn't mean much, and **free-range**, which means the chicken has access to the outdoors, though the actual amount of access is so limited it might make us cringe. And as always, we prefer **organic**, to avoid hormones and antibiotics.

SEAFOOD

LOOK FOR: Wild, MSC Certified, and Sustainable

The landscape of our vast, amazing oceans can be difficult to grasp. And then, we hear of things like mercury, soy pellets, extinction, and precious dolphins caught in tuna nets. How do we eat seafood without feeling guilty? And yet, seafood provides a supreme powerhouse of nutrition, serving as a staple for many traditional diets.

We choose to eat seafood, but as with our land-based meats, we do not take that decision lightly—and we've learned a few tricks along the way to help guide us, such as "the big fish eat the little fish" perspective, which reminds us that if we eat the little fish, we eat a lesser accumulation of mercury. If nothing else, that perspective has caused us to open our minds to lovely fish such as sardines (delicious chopped and tossed in Simply Mayonnaise, page 178) and anchovies (perfect in Caesar Salad with Sourdough Croutons, page 106). We also choose **wild seafood** because we have yet to learn of fish-farming practices that feel healthy and sustainable, and in navigating our wild seafood, we turn to an organization called the **Marine Stewardship Council, or MSC** (page 216), a certification and labeling program for sustainable seafood. When MSC certification is unavailable or unknown, **Seafood Watch** (see Resources, page 216), a program run by the Monterey Bay Aquarium, offers printable pocket guides and a searchable online database that outline the sustainability of each species. Many of our favorite recipes, such as Fresh Herb–Crusted Sea Bass with Sourdough Bread Crumbs (page 118) must be reevaluated when MSC-certified fish is unavailable.

PORK

LOOK FOR: Local, Pastured, Certified Humane, and Organic

If you can believe it, pigs are actually very clean creatures. They use mud to cool themselves down, not because living in mud is their top choice. Ideally, pigs prefer wooded areas, where they can roam freely or be moved frequently using portable fences. In the areas of the United States where woodland is unavailable, pigs at least prefer quality space, appropriate shade and sun, clean water, and ample fresh food. These days, however, many factory-farmed pigs live a tightly confined life in temperature-controlled buildings with concrete floors, likely covered in feces. Sad, isn't it?

Lucky for the pigs, and us, there are small- to medium-size pig farmers across the United States who think pigs need room to roam, too. As always, the number one place to begin the search for a compassionate farmer is at a local farmers' market, but because quality **pastured** pork can be slightly more difficult to source than its beef and poultry counterparts, you may also find it more convenient to order online; see Resources (page 216) for a listing of quality pastured pork that can be shipped to your home. When navigating a grocery store, I choose pork products that carry the label **Certified Humane** (an organization that will change the landscape of factory farming around the world) and **organic** (to avoid hormones and antibiotics).

Simply cooked chicken, bless its humble self, shows up in so many recipes and in the most delightful ways. There's chicken soup, chicken salad, chicken pot pie ... you get my drift. We'd like to show you a simple, foolproof recipe guaranteed to precook chicken in a moist and tasty fashion every time. It's called for in some favorite recipes in the book, including our White Bean Chicken Chili (page 96) and The New Poppy Seed Chicken Casserole (page 127).

Basic Precooked Chicken

Chicken breasts, split, bone-in,
  skin on
Sea salt

**YIELD: 1 CUP (140 G) CHOPPED
CHICKEN PER HALF BREAST**

RECIPE NOTE

Chilling the cooled, de-boned meat before chopping or shredding allows for a more uniform prep.

Place the chicken breasts in a suitably sized stockpot. A 6-quart (5.4 L) pot works well for 4 pieces (2 large breasts, split). Fill the pot with enough purified water to thoroughly cover the meat. Add ¼ teaspoon salt for each half breast. This ratio applies no matter how much chicken you cook.

Over high heat, bring the water to a full boil. Cover and lower the heat enough to maintain a nice steady simmer without allowing the liquid to boil over, about medium-high heat. If scum appears on top of the liquid, skim it off with a spoon and cover again. Continue cooking until a paring knife slides easily into the thickest part of the breast. This time will vary depending on the size and number of the breasts being cooked. On average, the total cook time will be about 15 minutes *after a boil is reached*, plus about 5 additional minutes per half breast. (Example: For 4 half breasts, the approximate cook time would be 35 minutes, or 15 minutes + 5 minutes + 5 minutes + 5 minutes + 5 minutes.) Once the desired tenderness is achieved, turn off the heat and let the chicken rest in the hot broth, covered, for 30 minutes.

After 30 minutes, remove the lid and allow the chicken to cool completely submerged in the broth. Removing the meat before it is cooled sacrifices the moist quality of this method.

Once cooled, remove the meat and discard the broth. Place the meat on a large-size platter where the skin and bones can easily be removed with your fingers. At this point you can refrigerate the cooked, de-boned chicken in a sealed container or prep as desired for any recipe.

Nitrates, a common additive in bacon that is used to prevent botulism during the curing process, are controversial because of their negative effect on health. Regardless of your individual stance on this matter, some people are indeed sensitive to them and must find an alternative. The good news is that nitrate-free bacon is available from local, small farmers or online (page 216). Beware of bacon that advertises "no nitrates added," but lists celery juice or powder in the ingredients, because this is just a natural substitute for powdered nitrates. Even though it is natural, a nitrate is a nitrate to the body, and must be avoided by those who have this sensitivity.

Oven-Roasted Bacon and Bacon Fat

1 pound (454 g) bacon

YIELD: 14 TO 16 STRIPS BACON, PLUS ½ CUP (120 ML) OR MORE BACON FAT

Preheat the oven to 350ºF (180ºC, or gas mark 4). Have ready 2 baking trays and 2 cooling racks. Place 1 cooling rack inside each baking tray. Lay the bacon in a single layer on top of the racks; the tray underneath will be used to catch the drippings.

Bake for 35 to 40 minutes, until the bacon is slightly crispy, but not burnt. Less crispy bacon prevents the oils from charring. Transfer the bacon to a plate.

Allow the trays to cool to the touch, but before the fat/drippings solidify, carefully scrape them into a glass container, straining if desired. Store bacon fat at room temperature and use to sauté vegetables or fry eggs; we also call for it in several recipes in this book. If not used up within a couple of weeks, transfer to the fridge for longer storage (ours never seems to make it there!).

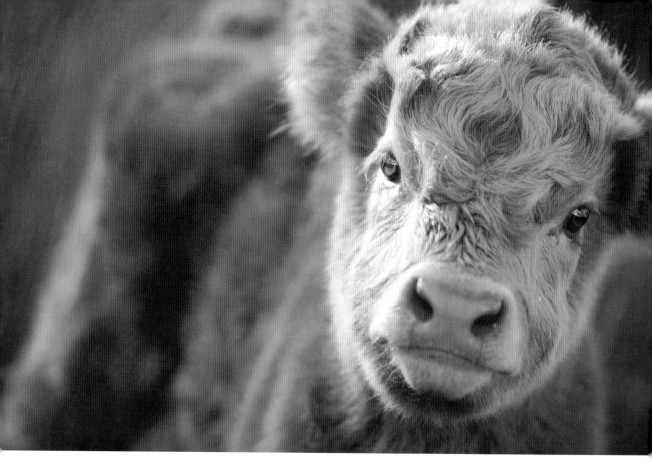

DAIRY

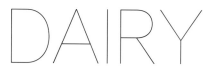

TO EACH HIS OWN

Food is so personal. When I was nine years old, on a low-key Friday night, my mom, Sandy, ordered a pizza with pepperoni, and when it arrived, I explained that I wouldn't be eating that pizza because "I am a vegetarian." To which my brother responded, "Yeah, right." But I was—for the next eighteen years. The reason? My only recollection is having a super-cool vegetarian friend teach me that an egg was a baby chicken. I ended up eating eggs anyway, and dairy, too, but back then, dairy most likely meant Velveeta, so I use the term loosely. Although I obviously wasn't living a healthy version of the lifestyle, I believe you can sustain and build health with a vegetarian diet, assuming there's an understanding of high-quality dairy products.

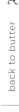

But what about a vegan diet, where no animal fats or proteins whatsoever are consumed? Although I realize my position is controversial, I do not believe it is possible to be vegan and build the health of future generations. Short-term cleansing? Yes. Can a strong body be sustained for a lifetime? Possibly, but not several generations of health. I also challenge the wisdom behind requiring a growing fetus or child to be vegan. Over time, the body suffers when vegetable proteins and fats are considered an equal substitute for animal proteins and fats. It is not uncommon for children raised under these paradigms to suffer from early and rampant dental cavities, a symptom of internal weakness.

However, I also support the individual's right to arrive at his or her own conclusions. Although I now eat animal fats and proteins, I look back on my time as a vegetarian with respect because it ultimately led me to understanding more about the quality farming and animal husbandry I practice today.

DAIRY DECISIONS

Regardless of whether or not we choose to eat animals, we should know the quality of the soil in which our vegetables, grains, and legumes were grown. And folks, it will take the assistance of animals and their manure to maintain it. If we eat animals, we need to understand how that animal was raised and with what diet. We must be careful not to force our personal choices on Mother Nature and her plants and animals.

Animals are naturally carnivores, omnivores, or herbivores, and to change their diet based on personal human beliefs is cruel. Which brings us to dairy cows. My friends—cows are vegans. They can't subsist on sugar (grain)—they need greens (grass). Let's take a minute to understand what *grass-fed* means, along with a few other important farming and milk-processing buzzwords.

GRASS-FED

As mentioned, cows are naturally grass-eating herbivores, and we must allow our animals the space to roam and forage. Honoring these natural instincts results in nutrient-dense milk products, such as the ones described by Dr. Weston A. Price (page 11–12). This same rule applies to all milked animals, including sheep and goats, who also prefer a side of weeds and brush with their grass. To sustain the energy that cows need to consistently produce milk, however, all dairy cows receive supplemental grain—the key word being *supplemental*.

There are reputable organizations regulating the certification of grass-based farming, including the American Grassfed Association and the U.S. Department of Agriculture (USDA). However, at this point, these regulations are still relatively new and evolving. Therefore, it is our opinion that the best grass-fed "certification" is getting to know your farmers and their practices.

> **"The fat within dairy aids digestion of the vitamins and minerals in the milk, which is why it's important to choose whole milk over its lower-fat counterparts."**

ORGANIC

Under the USDA definition of *organic agriculture*, farmers with this certification do not use preventive hormones or antibiotics to maintain herd health. Many quality grass-based farmers, however, do not take on the added expense and paperwork to achieve organic certification. In this understandable circumstance, it is simply important to ask your farmers about their perspective on chemical use, in order to ensure their philosophy mirrors your own.

WHOLE FAT

I can remember back when my mom began buying skim milk. My brother and I hated it, and honestly, I think we were on to something. The low-fat and nonfat trend has pervaded every inch of our culture, and it is thankfully *beginning* to retreat. The fat within dairy aids digestion of the vitamins and minerals in the milk, which is why it's important to choose whole milk over its lower-fat counterparts. Plus, fat fills us up, rendering between-meal snacking virtually unnecessary. Case in point: In 2005, the Harvard School of Public Health published a study examining weight and milk consumption of more than 12,000 U.S. children aged nine to fourteen years old. Researchers found that "contrary to our hypotheses, dietary calcium and skim and 1 percent milk were associated with weight gain, but dairy fat was not."

PASTEURIZATION

Pasteurization is the controversial method of heating milk to a minimum of 162°F (72°C) for 15 seconds in the attempt to kill pathogens. Ultra-pasteurization goes even further, and is a process that heats milk almost instantaneously to 280°F (138°C), which seems extreme. In the process of heating milk, many of the milk enzymes (lactase) that actually help the body digest milk sugar (lactose) are destroyed. As a result, it is fairly common for a lactose-intolerant person to be able to digest grass-fed, untreated milk. Regardless of your family's decision on this matter, pasteurization should not be used as a substitute for poor farming practices. Please read the sidebar "What Happened to My Milk?" (page 38) for further discussion.

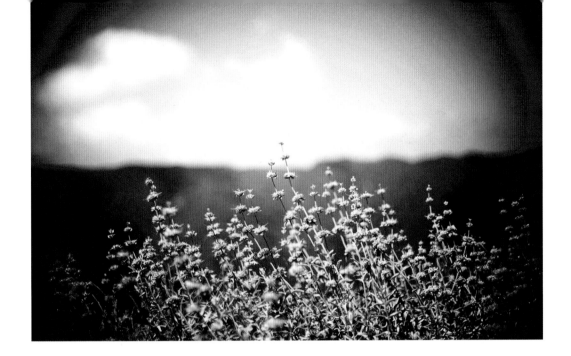

HOMOGENIZATION

Milk straight from the cow, when left undisturbed, naturally separates into milky water topped by fatty cream. Homogenization is a mechanical process of spinning the milk at such a high velocity that it breaks down the fat molecules into smaller particles so that the milk no longer separates. The purpose is largely for aesthetics and functionality, and there is controversy over the impact of the smaller protein molecules on our digestive system. Given that Mom and I don't mind giving a bottle of milk a shake before pouring a glass, and consider it a safer option, we always choose nonhomogenized.

RAW

Raw milk is any milk that has not been treated by pasteurization or homogenization. It comes straight from the cow and is loaded with natural digestive enzymes. When choosing raw, the health of the animal and the careful practices of the farmer are critical. Get to know your farmer! All milk was sold raw in the United States before routine pasteurization began in the 1920s. To utilize the beneficial enzymes, you'll see that we use quality raw milk products for all dairy recipes that are unheated, such as our Homemade Milk Kefir, Homemade Whole Milk Buttermilk, and Homemade Crème Fraîche (pages 42–45).

IN SUMMARY

Sometimes in the grocery store aisles, navigating milk products feels difficult and complicated. Therefore, to simplify this process, we suggest you locate and purchase milk products from a responsible, grass-based farmer. More often than not, the milk they sell is grass-fed, organic, whole-fat, unpasteurized, nonhomogenized, old-fashioned … raw milk.

"WHAT HAPPENED TO MY MILK?"

by Sandy Schrecengost

As a kid, I never analyzed milk. I just drank it. Big words like *pasteurized* and *homogenized* meant nothing to me. I loved milk, fired straight from the cow by my grandpa, or scooped from the milk house cooler in the heat of summer.

How times have changed. It's no longer easy—and in some states even illegal—to buy raw milk. Even the term *raw* is new. Milk just used to be milk; now it's heated and treated and stuffed with additives and antibiotics. Make no mistake, Molly and I support safe, healthy farming practices. Animals carry pathogens. We get that. Consequently, cows need to get to pasture and their spaces must be clean. Farm sanitation isn't something to be taken lightly. Yet it turns out some of these genuine attempts to ensure safe milk are complicating that effort and diminishing nutrition in the process.

The downside of such a broad stroke like pasteurization is that while it can be helpful, it can also be harmful. The high-heat processing destroys the healthy enzymes and beneficial bacteria which are present in raw milk and critical for digestion and assimilation of dairy. Pasteurization also significantly alters the very make-up of milk by altering the milk protein, and even diminishing milk's inherit vitamin content (see www.westonaprice.org). This kind of processing ultimately puts Nature's wisdom up against man's ever-changing knowledge.

When farm practices are healthy and the inherent needs of the animal are respected, consuming raw milk holds great advantage over processed milk. A study published in the highly respected journal *Lancet* showed raw milk reduces tooth decay—even in kids who eat sugar. A study published by Ohio State University showed that raw milk also promotes calcium absorption, which is so important amid the challenges of osteoporosis, and also results in far less allergic skin issues. But a staggering reason to consider raw over pasteurized is asthma. This unfortunate condition is reaching frightening proportions in our own nation's children. Yet another *Lancet* study showed that raw milk consumption greatly reduces a child's chances for developing asthma. Clearly, a seemingly simple question— "What kind of milk to buy?"—is no longer simple. It's critical.

The process of pasteurization was put in place to provide safe milk. Yet, consider this: If an animal is raised honoring its innate needs and treated with ancient wisdom and respect, the milk produced by that animal is already safe. It has been for centuries. So why mess with the milk? Shouldn't our focus go back to safe farming instead of indiscriminately overcompensating for unhealthy farm practices?

It seems evident to us that the benefits of raw milk outweigh the risk. The United States is among a small list of countries in the world that aggressively regulate milk. Canada joins us. Yet the majority of the countries in Europe and Asia sell raw milk without governmental regulation. New Zealand, in our humble opinion, seems to handle this issue most logically. This country highly regulates raw milk production to offset pathogen risk, permitting raw milk to be sold directly from the producer/farm only. Rather than throw the amazing health benefits out with the broad stroke of government regulation, New Zealand has found a way to allow its citizens to assume responsibility of choice while maintaining product quality and nutrition—by knowing their farmers!

This book isn't a poster child for raw milk. We recognize such a choice holds a risk only you can decide to embrace or decline. We sincerely respect that. All food carries risk. Wisdom should be the first tool in your consumer pocket, and we should all have the right to choose either product. *Legally.* It's not our intent to dictate what you eat, how you source food, or even how you prepare it. We simply believe raw or pasteurized should be a choice.

To you, safe milk with maximum nutrition might mean pasteurized. To us, it means raw. Yet, in order to reduce the risk of raw milk, we want to know our farmer and his livestock practices firsthand. Because no matter what choice we make, all milk should come from a healthy animal that's been treated humanely.

This recipe begins with yogurt, which we strain and separate into a tangy, versatile cream cheese, used for delights like Cultured Cream Cheese Olive Dip (page 73), and whey, a liquid by-product that holds its own uses and benefits.

Real whey, obtained from yogurt or milk, contains an abundance of naturally occurring probiotics, which are the healthy bacteria that live in our gut and keep unhealthy bacteria in check. It's funny that some people pay hard-earned money for vitamins filled with freeze-dried probiotics, when eating fermented foods produces the same effect (if not greater), for a fraction of the price! The "live" nature of whey also means that it can be used to activate fermentation in cultured foods, so be sure to keep a jar stored in your refrigerator for that purpose alone. It's also great for soaking beans and grains (see next chapter).

Yogurt Cream Cheese and Whey

1 quart (1 L) whole milk yogurt

YIELD: 2 CUPS (470 ML) WHEY AND 1½ CUPS (345 G) CREAM CHEESE

Set a fine-mesh strainer over a large-size (2-quart [1.8 L] or larger) nonmetal bowl and line the strainer with a thin tea towel. Using a thin cloth is important to allow the liquid to seep through.

Pour the yogurt into the lined strainer. Cover the strainer with a lid or plate and set aside at room temperature for 4 to 6 hours. If your house is exceptionally warm (above 80ºF [27ºC]), place this whole setup in the fridge. Check occasionally to see if the whey has stopped dripping into the bowl; once it has, or the 4 to 6 hours is up, move on to the next step. The yogurt at this point will resemble Greek yogurt (which it is!).

When the drips subside, remove the cover, place a wooden spoon across the mesh strainer, and double-knot the diagonal corners of the tea towel over the top of the spoon handle. Set a tall container, such as a wide-mouth vase or pitcher, next to the strainer. Carefully lift the knotted tea towel and lower it into the tall vessel, allowing the spoon handle to rest on the rim of the vessel. The tea towel should be a few inches (cm)

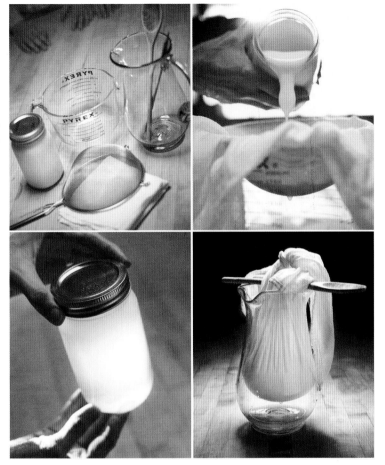

CLOCKWISE, FROM TOP LEFT: Equipment setup; pouring yogurt into the strainer; straining additional whey, final jar of whey

from the bottom of the container, so it doesn't mingle with any resulting whey. Be careful not to squeeze the towel. It should drip slowly on its own.

Pour the whey from the bottom of the original bowl into a glass jar or container with a tight-fitting lid and store in the fridge for future use. Place the vessel/spoon/tea towel operation into the fridge as well, and allow it to continue dripping for 8 to 12 hours or overnight. It is finished when the dripping stops and the yogurt "cream cheese" feels firm.

After whey stops dripping, remove the tea towel and place on a cutting board. Add the remaining whey to your jar of whey from the day before. Untie the tea towel from the wooden spoon. Scrape the cream cheese into a glass bowl with a tight-fitting lid and use like any store-bought cream cheese. We think it's just perfect in our Maple Walnut Cake with Maple Cream Cheese Frosting (page 203). Keep in mind that it will have a yogurt sweetness but with a bit of tang.

Kept refrigerated, the cream cheese will last for about 1 month and the whey up to 6 months.

Kefir is a fermented dairy beverage that is slightly thinner than yogurt and a bit zestier. Due to the fermentation it undergoes, kefir is an extremely probiotic-rich food. Think of a glass of kefir as your daily dose of Nature's antibiotics. Kefir also feeds off the lactose in the milk, which lowers the overall amount of lactose in the beverage and may be tolerated more easily by those who are generally lactose intolerant. If choosing to try this, please use caution and begin slowly. Lactose intolerance is case specific and not to be taken lightly.

The first step of making kefir is sourcing kefir grains (page 216, or a friend with excess if you're so lucky). The grain pictured on page 43, looks a bit like tiny cauliflower florets and can be reused with each batch. If you choose to use raw milk, we encourage researching a safe source to procure it (page 216). Once these two items are on hand, along with a jar with a *plastic* lid (as metal is reactive and may cause an off taste), making kefir is a cinch! Enjoy it in fruit smoothies; use it as you would buttermilk; or strain it following the same method as our Yogurt Cream Cheese and Whey (page 40), mix in some herbs and salt, and indulge in some deliciously tangy kefir cheese.

Homemade Milk Kefir

½ cup (96 g) hydrated kefir grains

3 cups (705 ml) nonhomogenized whole milk, preferably raw

YIELD: 3 CUPS (704 ML)

In a 1-quart (1 L) Mason jar, combine the kefir grains and milk. Put on a plastic lid (no need to seal tightly) and leave at room temperature (72ºF [22ºC]) for 12 hours.

After 12 hours, remove the lid and use a clean spoon to taste and check the texture. The taste should be sour, yet pleasant, and the texture should have thickened slightly to a very thin yogurt. If the kefir is not ready, replace the lid and set aside for an additional 6 hours. If still not ready, return the lid and set aside for another 6 hours, repeating until the proper consistency is attained.

Depending on the vitality of the grains and the temperature of the room, fermentation times can vary. It may take up to 24 to 36 hours. If you want to speed the process with future batches, begin with more grains and/or less milk, and set the jar in a warmer location. If the kefir ferments too quickly, resulting in a taste that is too sour, cut back on the amount of kefir grains and/or place the jar in a cooler location. As with most things, it takes some practice, but it's worth it!

Once ready, place a strainer on top of a large-size, nonmetal bowl and pour the kefir and kefir grains into the strainer. Use a rubber spatula to gently stir the grains, allowing the liquid kefir to strain into the bowl and the kefir grains to remain in the strainer. Once all the liquid kefir has been strained, return the grains to the jar, along with fresh milk. Pour the liquid kefir in the bowl into a clean Mason jar, seal, and store in the fridge until you're ready to use.

JUST SAY NO TO ULTRAPASTEURIZED

If you cannot source raw milk in your area or are more comfortable with grocery store alternatives, be sure to buy *pasteurized* and not *ultrapasteurized* milk, as the latter is heated to such a high temperature that it is essentially dead and cannot be used to culture kefir, buttermilk, cream, or the like. Keep in mind, even organic milk from the grocery store is often ultrapasteurized.

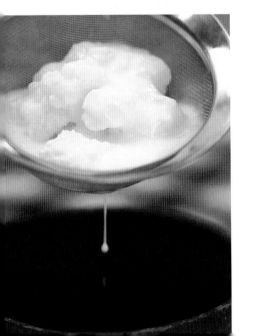

RECIPE NOTES

• If you want to take a break from the kefir process for any reason, simply place a freshly prepared jar of kefir grains and milk in the refrigerator. The grains will last for two weeks in the fridge and two months or more in the freezer. When you want to resume, simply defrost (if necessary), strain the kefir grains as described above, and discard the milk. Rinse the grains to remove the soured milk, and then proceed as above. Note that the first few cycles of kefir may not develop to your taste (a necessary evil of vacationing!). If this happens, discard the milk and start again. Eventually, the grains will produce as expected.

• Kefir also can be made using powdered packets (page 216). The benefit of fresh kefir grains over powdered is their ability to continue culturing for years, because they typically contain more diverse strains of probiotics than the powdered version. Powdered packets are beneficial for people who frequently travel because after three or four batches of kefir, a new packet must be used. When ordering packets of kefir, follow the simple instructions that come with the box.

• Plastic Mason jar lids are often found along with canning materials at your local hardware store, or may be ordered online. They're perfect for storing kefir and other ferments.

Store-bought buttermilk is often low in quality and supplemented with milk powder, which is a perfect reason to try making it at home! The process could not be simpler. First, order a few buttermilk cultures (page 216), then culture away. This culture-rich liquid is a versatile ingredient capable of bringing added moisture to baked goods, a nice tang to a batch of pancakes, or a delightful texture to creamy salad dressings.

Homemade Whole Milk Buttermilk

1 quart (1 L) nonhomogenized
   whole milk, preferably raw
1 packet powdered buttermilk
   culture

YIELD: 1 QUART (1 L)

In a small-size pot over medium-low heat, warm the milk to 85° to 90°F (29° to 32°C). If you don't have a thermometer handy, simply place a drop of milk on the inside of your wrist, right below your palm. The milk should not feel cool or hot. When appropriately heated, remove the pan from the heat.

Stir the buttermilk culture into the milk until fully dissolved and pour into a 1-quart (1 L) Mason jar. Put on the lid and leave at room temperature for 12 to 24 hours, until thickened. Once thickened, refrigerate and use as needed. Buttermilk will last for at least 1 week in the fridge.

Crème fraîche is a luxurious, European-style sour cream that is really easy to make at home, where the cook controls the quality of the ingredients. It's a bit thicker and slightly less sour than American sour cream, making it a perfect dessert topping. The texture and flavor also work perfectly in our Millet Salmon Cakes with Creamy Dipping Sauce (page 116). Raw cream works great in this recipe; however, we encourage researching a safe source to procure it (page 216).

Homemade Crème Fraîche

1½ cups (355 ml) heavy cream,
   preferably raw
1 tablespoon (15 ml) buttermilk
   (page 44)

YIELD: 1½ CUPS (355 ML)

In a pint-size (470 ml) Mason jar, combine the cream and buttermilk and stir well. Place the lid on the jar and leave at room temperature (the warmer the better) for 24 hours, or until thickened. Stir the cream and refrigerate; it will continue to thicken as it chills. Crème fraîche will last for several weeks in the refrigerator, and can also be whisked into whipped cream the same way as regular heavy cream.

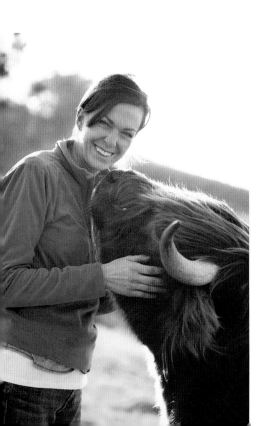

The preceding dairy recipes in this chapter do not heat the milk to high temperatures; therefore, if you have chosen to source raw milk for your family, they are excellent applications for it. However, when a recipe calls for heating the milk, as does the creamy cheese sauce below, some of the benefits of raw milk are actually lost in the cooking process, so it's equally nutritious to use grass-fed, nonhomogenized, organic milk and cream (but never ultra-pasteurized!). Be sure to try this recipe with our Baked Potatoes with the Works (page 124), which is a family favorite.

Foolproof Cheese Sauce

3 tablespoons (42 g) butter

2 tablespoons (16 g) arrowroot powder

2 cups (470 ml) whole milk

1 cup (235 ml) cream

2 cups (240 g) grated white Cheddar cheese

1 teaspoon sea salt

¼ teaspoon freshly cracked white pepper

¼ teaspoon freshly grated nutmeg

⅛ teaspoon crushed red pepper flakes

In a medium-size saucepan over medium heat, melt the butter until foaming. Add the arrowroot and whisk well until combined. Slowly add the milk and cream, whisking constantly, until lightly simmering, about 5 minutes. The mixture should thicken slightly due to the arrowroot.

Remove from the heat. Add the cheese, whisking constantly, until fully melted. Stir in the sea salt, pepper, nutmeg, and red pepper flakes. Serve warm.

YIELD: 1¾ CUPS (411 ML)

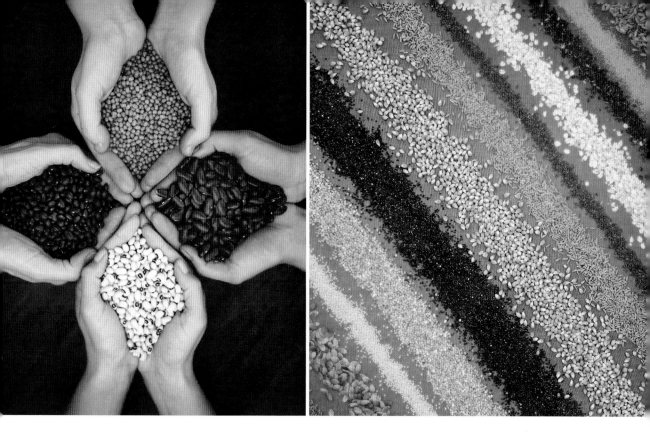

CHAPTER 4

NUTS, SEEDS, BEANS & GRAINS

WHY ALL THE SPECIAL TREATMENT?

One of the major differences between the diet of traditional cultures and the modern diets of today is the treatment of grains, legumes/beans, nuts, and seeds. In traditional cultures, if these foods were included in the diet at all, they were carefully soaked, sprouted, or soured/fermented, such as in our Rustic Sourdough Bread (page 186) or Chester Cookies (page 196). Today, these methods have largely fallen by the wayside, and unfortunately so.

> "Examples of an acidic medium for soaking, which we refer to in our recipes as an 'activator,' are kombucha, whey, and lemon juice."

The primary reason behind all the special treatment of yesteryear is, in fact, rooted in science. Although our ancestors may not have used the terms *enzyme inhibitors* and *phytic acid*, these anti-nutrients, found in grains, beans, nuts, and seeds, prevent us from digesting these foods properly or getting the most out of them nutritionally—unless their effects are mitigated by **soaking** (with an acidic medium), **sprouting**, or **souring/fermenting**. Such treatment methods break down those nasty anti-nutrients, thereby making the foods easier to digest and more nourishing.

PHYTIC ACID AND ENZYME INHIBITORS, DEFINED

- **Enzyme inhibitors** are molecules that bind to the healthy digestive and metabolic enzymes in our body, rendering them useless and inhibiting our digestive power.
- **Phytic acid** is a plant's principal storage of phosphorus—which would be great, if we could digest it. We can't, though, and even more troublesome, phytic acid renders micronutrients, including zinc, iron, magnesium, and calcium, useless.

If one or more of the treatment methods mentioned above is not followed, the two irritants can cause digestive issues (due to improper digestion/absorption). Over the years, I have known folks who could not tolerate any nuts in their diet, until they began soaking them. Pretty powerful! But be aware that the effectiveness of this technique can be inadequate when dealing with extreme allergies to nuts, so use caution and personal discretion. Likewise, many people who are irritated by grains have no trouble digesting authentic sourdough bread, because the grains/flours have been "predigested," if you will, by fermentation.

The technique recipes that follow outline just what you need to do to get started, and can be used for just about any nut, seed, or grain. Examples of an acidic medium for soaking, which we refer to in our recipes as an "activator," are kombucha, whey, and lemon juice. Although all of these techniques take time, it's mostly hands-off and the end result should make a world of difference in how you feel. I'm guessing traditional cultures didn't know a thing about anti-nutrients in the technical sense, but instinct led them to these answers—and it is to the benefit of our universal health to keep these practices alive today.

The following soaking and drying instructions work for all nuts and seeds except cashews. Cashews, which actually aren't raw when they reach us anyway, can get slimy if soaked too long and are best limited to a 6-hour soak time. Nuts such as pecans, almonds, walnuts, and hazelnuts, however, all process well with this technique, as do seeds of just about any kind, except flax and chia seeds, which turn gelatinous when soaked (making them great for baking, but not for straining and dehydrating). Finally, keep in mind that the high oil content of nuts requires freezing for storage, if they are not consumed within a few days.

Soaking & Drying Technique: Crunchy Nuts and Seeds

Inspired by Sally Fallon

4 cups (580 g) raw nuts or seeds

2 tablespoons (30 ml) whey

1 tablespoon (18 g) sea salt, plus more to taste

YIELD: 4 CUPS (580 G)

NOT ALL WATER IS CREATED EQUAL

In all of our recipes where water is called for soaking/fermenting, we recommend using filtered or purified water because chemicals and contaminants in tap water (like chlorine) can interfere with the soaking and absorption process.

In a large-size glass bowl, combine the nuts, whey, sea salt, and enough room-temperature water to cover the nuts by 2 inches (5 cm). Stir to dissolve the salt. Cover with a lid or plate and set in a warm place, approximately 75ºF (24ºC), for 24 hours.

Once the soaking is complete, set your oven or food dehydrator to 150ºF (66ºC). Rinse the nuts well in a colander (discard the soaking water) and spread in a single layer onto regular sheet pans or dehydrator trays with mesh inserts. Sprinkle lightly with sea salt, to taste (feel free to try a few!).

Dry in the oven or dehydrator for 12 to 24 hours. Most nuts take only 12 to 15 hours, but almonds and hazelnuts almost always take a full 24 and even up to 36 hours. The nuts are ready when they crunch nicely upon biting, with no residual moisture. Always test several nuts to ensure uniform dehydration.

Store nuts in an airtight container in the freezer or refrigerator.

Store-bought nut butters are typically made from nuts that have not been soaked. Making them at home allows you to create a delicious soaked version, while also controlling the quality of the sea salt and oils that are added for taste and texture.

Soaked Almond Butter

3 cups (about 1 pound, or 454 g) crunchy almonds (page 49)

2 tablespoons (28 g) unrefined coconut oil

Sea salt, to taste

YIELD: 3 CUPS (454 G)

Optional First Step: Preheat the oven to 350°F (180°C, or gas mark 4). On a large-size sheet tray, spread the almonds in a single layer. Bake for 10 minutes, until fragrant and lightly browned. Set aside to cool completely.

If you like your almond butter crunchy, remove ½ cup (65 g) of almonds, roughly chop, and set aside. Place the remaining almonds into the bowl of a food processor. Turn on the motor and process for 1 minute; the almonds will be grainy.

Add the oil and salt, and restart the motor. After a few minutes, the almond butter will turn into a ball. After a few more minutes, it will separate from the ball and stick to the sides of the bowl. Finally, it will become smooth. The whole process takes about 5 minutes. Once smooth, if making crunchy almond butter, add the chopped almonds back to the bowl and pulse briefly until combined. Scoop into an airtight container and refrigerate. The almond butter will thicken slightly when refrigerated.

NOT ALL BEANS ARE CREATED EQUAL

Soy contains estrogenlike properties that could negatively affect you or even your babies. It certainly compromised my health for many years, causing my cycles to extend to forty-five days or more, my face to dramatically break out, and cysts to appear on my ovaries. It's serious and something worth looking into if you are (or were) a soy consumer. Could I have changed my fate by eliminating soy? All I know is that those symptoms were completely gone three months after removing soy from my diet.

Unlike with tofu and other highly processed soy products, however, many people find that *traditionally fermented* soy works well for their bodies. These foods, including tempeh, miso, natto, and naturally brewed soy sauce, are prepared with the wisdom of traditional cultures and have merit. We simply encourage awareness that soy may not live up to the hype for all bodies.

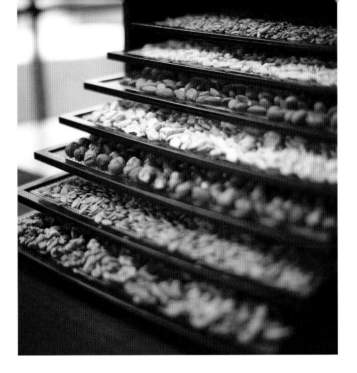

THE LOWDOWN ON DEHYDRATORS

My first time working with dehydrators was back in culinary school, while intern-ing at a popular raw foods restaurant, and I've loved them ever since.

Dehydrators are small, mobile ovens that dry food at very low temperatures, usually ranging from 90° to 160°F (32° to 71°C). Pure "raw foodists," who are after the preservation of enzyme content, typically prefer keeping the temperature somewhere below 120°F (49°C), but because I am more concerned with removing phytic acid and enzyme inhibitors—and because I prefer the aesthetic "crunch" provided by a slightly higher dehydration temperature—I stick with 150°F (66°C) for grains, nuts, and seeds.

Dehydrators can also be used for a variety of other foods and are excellent for preserving summer's bounty (dried apricots, anyone?). Here are some common dehydration temperatures we suggest:

Fruit Leathers: 115°F (46°C)

Sun-Dried Tomatoes: 125°F (52°C)

Dried Fruit: 125°F (52°C)

Sprouted Grains, Nuts, and Seeds: 150°F (66°C)

Meat Jerky: 130° to 170°F (54° to 77°C)

As we've said, beans contain properties that actually prevent our bodies from absorbing the minerals in our foods. The good news is that proper preparation, including a long soak and a slow cooking process, neutralizes those destructive properties, restoring beans to their healthy status. If needed, this recipe is easily doubled.

Soaking & Cooking Technique: Beans

1 cup (250 g) dried black beans, kidney beans, pinto beans, black-eyed peas, chickpeas, or white beans

2 tablespoons (30 ml) activator, such as plain kombucha (page 209), whey (page 40), or lemon juice

7 cups (1.65 L) water

1 piece (3 inches, or 7.5 cm) of kombu

2 teaspoons sea salt

YIELD: 2 TO 3 CUPS (344 TO 515 G)

RECIPE NOTES

• Even for a single batch, kidney beans and chickpeas benefit from doubling the amount of activator used for soaking because they have a tougher exterior.

• Kombu (page 217) is a type of dried seaweed that imparts additional minerals and flavor into the cooking liquid, along with beneficial enzymes, which help break down the sugars in the bean.

Put the beans in a glass container with a lid and cover with warm water by 2 inches (5 cm). Stir in the activator, cover, and leave in a warm place 12 to 36 hours. Longer soaking removes additional phytic acid; if soaking longer than 12 hours, however, change the water and activator every 12 hours. After soaking, drain the beans and rinse well in a colander.

In a large-size heavy-bottomed pot, add the beans, the 7 cups fresh water, and the kombu. Bring to a boil, then reduce to a simmer, skimming off any foam that may have formed on the surface of the water with a large-size flat spoon. Cover the pot and simmer for 1½ to 4 hours; cooking time will depend on the type of bean, size, and age (older beans take longer to cook). When using beans for a salad, stop cooking once tender but before they lose their shape and become mushy.

Add sea salt toward the very end of the cooking process. When cooking is complete, remove the kombu (if small pieces of the kombu remain, don't worry about them). Store the beans in the refrigerator, in their cooking liquid, to use throughout the week. Drain and rinse as needed.

Millet and quinoa are two naturally gluten-free grains that are easy to soak and even easier to cook. Millet is one of the least allergenic and most easily digestible grains, with a somewhat nutty flavor and fluffy texture. Ever-popular quinoa is not really a grain at all, but rather a seed. It contains eight essential amino acids, and just 1 cup (185 g) provides 8 grams of protein! Note that there is a minimum of 25 hours of advance prep time.

Soaking & Cooking Technique: Millet & Quinoa

1 cup (173 g) millet or quinoa

6¾ cups (1585 ml) water, divided

4 tablespoons (60 ml) activator, such as plain kombucha (page 209), whey (page 40), or lemon juice, divided

¼ teaspoon sea salt

YIELD: 3 TO 4 CUPS (555 TO 740 G)

In a glass container with a lid, combine the millet, 3 cups (705 ml) of the water, and 2 tablespoons (30 ml) of the activator. Cover and set aside for 12 hours.

Pour the millet into a fine-mesh strainer and rinse well. Rinse the glass container. Return the millet to the container with 3 cups (705 ml) more fresh water and the remaining 2 table-spoons (30 ml) activator. Set aside for another 12 hours. Again, using a fine-mesh strainer, rinse the millet thoroughly.

In a small-size pot with a lid, bring the remaining ¾ cup (175 ml) water and sea salt to a boil. Once boiling, add the millet to the pot and stir once. Wait until the water returns to a boil, then cover and reduce the heat to low to maintain a gentle simmer. Set a timer for 10 minutes and don't peek!

After 10 minutes, lift the lid and check for liquid. To do so, push the handle of a wooden spoon straight down into the millet and pull along the bottom of the pot. If water appears, return the lid and cook in 2-minute increments until no water appears. Once done, replace the lid, turn off the heat, and allow to rest for 10 minutes, then fluff with a fork and serve (or refrigerate until needed).

The technique in this recipe may be used for all varieties of brown rice and even the unique red rice used in our Red Rice Salad with Cumin Dressing (page 109). Unlike white rice, brown and red rices are either unmilled or only partly milled, leaving the bran and the germ of the rice intact, and valuable vitamins and minerals untouched and available when prepared properly!

Soaking & Cooking Technique: Rice

1 cup (190 g) brown or red rice

6 cups (1410 ml) water, divided

4 tablespoons (60 ml) activator, such as plain kombucha (page 209), whey (page 40), or lemon juice, divided

2 cups (470 ml) homemade chicken stock (page 82)

¼ teaspoon sea salt

YIELD: 3⅓ CUPS (550 G)

In a glass container with a lid, combine the rice, 3 cups (705 ml) of the water, and 2 tablespoons (30 ml) of the activator. Cover and set aside for 12 hours.

Pour the rice into a fine-mesh strainer and rinse well. Rinse the glass container. Return the rice to the container with the remaining 3 cups (705 ml) fresh water and remaining 2 tablespoons (30 ml) activator. Set aside for another 12 hours. Again, using the fine-mesh strainer, rinse the rice thoroughly.

In a small-size pot with a lid over high heat, bring the chicken stock and sea salt to a boil. Once boiling, add the rinsed rice to the pot, stir once, and wait until the stock returns to a boil. Cover and reduce the heat to low to maintain a gentle simmer. Set a timer for 50 minutes and don't peek!

After 50 minutes, lift the lid and check for liquid. To do so, push the handle of a wooden spoon straight down into the rice and pull along the bottom of the pot. If water appears, return the lid and cook in 5-minute increments until no water appears. Once done, replace the lid, turn off the heat, and allow to rest for 10 minutes, then fluff with a fork and serve (or refrigerate until needed).

This technique can be used for all types of wheat berries, including spelt, einkorn, and kamut. The berries are soaked, sprouted, and dehydrated, then finally ground into what we refer to throughout the book as "fresh-milled, sprouted flour." We grind our berries using a residential mill grinder (page 217).

Soaking, Sprouting, Dehydrating, & Grinding Technique: Wheat

2 cups (140 g) wheat berries

YIELD: 2¼ CUPS (160 G)

Purchase or make a sprouting jar. To make it yourself, simply replace the lid of a 2-quart (2 L) Mason jar with mesh screening.

Add the wheat berries to the sprouting jar and fill the jar two-thirds full with water. Set aside, out of direct light, to soak for 8 hours, or overnight.

Drain off the soaking water and rinse the berries directly in the jar until foam subsides. Carefully tilt the jar to drain off the rinsing water, allowing the berries to disperse evenly along the full length of the jar.

Tilt the jar to a 45-degree angle, resting it in a dish rack or bowl. Make sure the mesh screen is not completely covered with berries to allow airflow into the jar, preventing mold. Make sure the angle ensures enough airflow into the screen.

Every 12 hours, rinse and drain the berries and return to position. After about 12 to 24 hours, the berries will begin to sprout. The berries need only grow tiny tails, as the best nutritional results (with grains) are achieved through minimal sprouting. At completion, the berries will look similar to an olive with a pimento barely sticking out (see photo on next page). Too long of a tail will cause issues with entering the mouth of the grain mill.

Once sprouted, rinse and drain one final time.

nuts, seeds, beans & grains

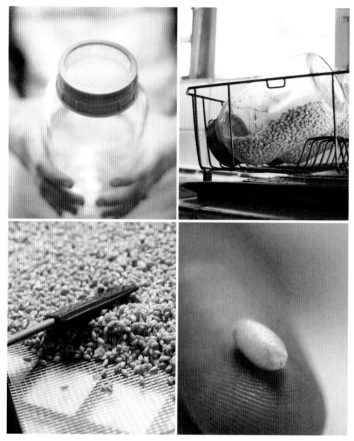

CLOCKWISE, FROM TOP LEFT: Sprouting jar with mesh lid; Dish rack set-up for airflow; Wheat berry with tiny sprout; Spreading sprouts to dry on dehydrator sheets

To prevent mold, the berries now need to be dried completely in a food dehydrator or an oven. Using a spatula, spread the berries ¼-inch (6 mm) thick on a dehydrator tray with a mesh insert or on a sheet pan if using an oven. Dry slowly at 150ºF (66ºC) for 12 to 24 hours. The berries are finished when they crunch when bitten. Cool completely before storing at room temperature in a sealed container.

Use a grain mill (page 217) to grind the dried berries into flour. Be sure to grind well; you're looking for a similar texture to that of store-bought whole wheat flour.

RECIPE NOTE

If drying your sprouted berries to grind into flour, keep in mind that the type of wheat used will change the end result. Hard red wheat berries yield bread flour; hard white wheat berries or golden 86 yield a lighter "all-purpose" flour; and soft white wheat berries yield pastry flour.

back to butter

In the beginnings of the summer on a breezy day, making a sourdough starter is pretty easy. But what about starting one in mid-winter? After many failed experiments in my kitchen, which stays cool year-round from Spanish tile, I decided I needed something to give the starter a jump-start. It was then that I glanced over at my kombucha ... success!

Sourdough Technique:
Rye Starter

Freshly milled (unsprouted) whole
  rye flour
Plain kombucha (page 209)

In the morning or evening, in a quart-size (1 L) Mason jar, combine ¼ cup (30 g) rye flour and ¼ cup (60 ml) kombucha. Stir until thoroughly combined. Cover the top with a cloth and set in a spot that is about 75ºF (24ºC); an oven with the light on and the door cracked works well.

Every 12 hours (morning and night) for 7 days, add ¼ cup (30 g) rye flour and ¼ cup (60 ml) kombucha to the jar and stir. Once the jar is halfway full, dump out half, then add the flour and kombucha. Do this each time it reaches this halfway point.

After 7 days, the starter should be bubbly and ready to use. Continue to feed the starter every 12 hours, discarding half before each feeding, but switch to water instead of kombucha. Once the starter is going strong, it can be kept in the fridge with a lid on it. Pull it out and feed it weekly when not in use, discarding half of the starter when necessary.

If your starter has been kept in the fridge for some time, pull it out a few days before you want to use it in a recipe. Keep it on the counter and feed morning and night with ¼ cup (30 g) rye flour and ¼ cup (60 ml) water for approximately 2 days, or until actively bubbly again.

Use recently fed starter in our Rustic Sourdough Bread recipe (page 186).

WHAT ABOUT CORN?

Corn contains vitamin B3, or niacin, but it is bound—meaning it cannot be absorbed—by our digestive system. Although they may not have referred to it as *niacin*, per say, Native Americans were aware of this absorption issue and learned to soak and cook their corn in ash water (an alkaline solution) to release this vitamin. The process, called nixtamalization, also helps prevent the horrible disease pellagra, caused by a chronic lack of niacin in the diet. The disease, which causes dementia, diarrhea, dermatitis, and more, underwent an outbreak in the South during the American Civil War, when poor farmworkers subsisted on unsoaked "quick cornmeal," unaware of the soaking and proper preparation correlation.

Although dried corn products are only eaten occasionally in the United States, it is still good practice to soak corn properly in an alkaline solution (such as ash, pickling lime, or baking soda) before grinding into cornmeal, the common term for all ground corn. Polenta and common American grits, two types of cornmeal on the market today, are not properly soaked and should therefore be used conservatively. Hominy grits and masa harina, on the other hand, are the soaked equivalents to polenta and cornmeal/flour. These are widely available, but are often not organic.

Fortunately for us, hominy, the basis for all other soaked corn products, can be made at home from dried corn, as described in the following recipe. The terminology in the world of corn is a bit complicated, however, so bear with me first for a quick overview. After **dried corn** gets an alkaline soak and a slow cook, the resulting puffy corn is known as **hominy** or **nixtamal**. **Fresh hominy** is used to make the dough for traditional corn tortillas; **dried hominy** is commonly used to make pozole, a delicious Mexican soup. When dried hominy is **coarsely** ground, it is called **hominy grits**, which is the equivalent of polenta, albeit properly treated; when dried hominy is *finely* ground, it is called **masa harina**, which is the equivalent to corn flour, but again properly treated. **Maize** is simply the Spanish word for corn that's now become commonplace in the United States as well.

CORN COMPREHENSION

TYPE OF CORN	UNTREATED	TREATED WITH ALKALINE SOLUTION
Whole Corn	Corn or Maize	Hominy (Fresh or Dried)
Coarsely Ground	Polenta/American Grits	Hominy Grits
Finely Ground	Cornmeal or Corn Flour	Masa Harina

Freshly cooked hominy is a wonderful substitute for pasta in soups and salads, or used as you would any bean. Although hominy can be made using several different alkaline solutions, including commercial lye, lye made from wood ash, pickling lime, or baking soda, we recommend pickling lime (also called cal or food-grade lime) because it is readily available, is safe and efficient, and leaves behind a clean-tasting hominy. Be sure to follow the instructions closely, especially the rinsing details, because lime is very alkaline and can mess with stomach acid if not properly rinsed. Note that this technique takes about 32 hours of preparation, though most of it is hands-off!

Soaking & Cooking Technique: Hominy

Inspired by Irv Kanode

½ cup (120 ml) pickling lime
   (page 217)
4 cups (540 g) dried corn

**YIELD: 11 CUPS (1725 G) FRESH OR
6 CUPS (840 G) DRIED**

In a large-size stainless steel or enamel-coated pot, add 5 quarts (4.5 L) of water and bring to a boil over high heat. Immediately upon boiling, turn off the heat, and stir in the lime using a wooden spoon, stirring until completely dispersed. Set aside to cool and settle for 5 hours, covered.

After 5 hours, the water will be almost clear with a layer of powdered lime resting on the bottom of the pot and a thin, crispy layer of lime coating the surface. Have ready another 7-quart (6.3 L) or larger enamel-coated pot, such as a Dutch oven, and rest a fine-mesh strainer across the top of the pot to catch the crispy layer (which you'll discard). Carefully pour the limewater through the strainer and into the clean pot without disturbing the powdered lime resting on the bottom. Stop pouring before the bulk of the powdered lime releases; this will result in about a cup or two of liquid left behind. A little bit of light powder may sneak into the pot, which is okay. If the lime powder stirs and causes too much liquid to be left behind, let the remainder settle again and rather than pouring, use a ladle to scoop off the last of the clear liquid.

Add the corn to the limewater in the clean pot, cover, and place in a room-temperature spot for 12 hours.

After soaking, preheat the oven to 250ºF (120ºC, or gas mark ½) and position the racks so that the pot can sit in the center of the oven. Over high heat, bring the covered limewater and corn to a boil. Keep a close eye on the pot, as you want to catch it right when it boils so that it doesn't boil over. As soon as it boils, turn off the heat and transfer the covered pot to the preheated oven for 2 hours.

After 2 hours, remove the pot from the oven. To test for doneness, use a slotted spoon to scoop several kernels into a fine-mesh strainer and run the strainer under cold water, until the kernels are cool and thoroughly rinsed. Bite into a kernel—it should seem cooked or al dente, without being hard. Test several before determining doneness, and return the pot to the hot oven for 15-minute increments until it reaches the desired tenderness.

Once cooked, carefully pour the kernels into a stainless steel colander and rinse with cool water for about a minute. Wash out the pot and return the kernels to it. Refill with cool, fresh water and set aside to soak for 5 minutes to remove any remaining lime. Strain once more through the colander and rinse for another minute, then drain.

Cooked hominy can be refrigerated for up to a week. It can also be frozen, but tends to be a bit mushy when thawed. To freeze, spread hominy in a single layer on a baking sheet and freeze. Once frozen, transfer the hominy to a container and store in the freezer for several months. If dried hominy is preferred, spread fresh hominy on the mesh inserts of dehydrator trays and dehydrate at 125ºF (52ºC) for 12 hours, or until the kernels are crisp throughout. Dried hominy can be stored in an airtight container at room temperature, and then ground into hominy grits or masa harina (see sidebar).

RECIPE NOTES

• Any type of whole, dried, non-GMO, organic corn, except popcorn, works for this recipe. Popcorn can work, but it doesn't plump up very nicely.

• The recipe calls for stainless steel or enamel-coated pots, which is an important step to follow. The lime can react with other types of pots and cause discoloration.

• Use an oven thermometer to ensure the oven temperature is accurate; too much heat can cause the kernels to over-cook and dissolve and too little heat can result in improperly cooked kernels.

HOW TO GRIND DRIED HOMINY

Dried, whole hominy can be finely or coarsely ground using a home grain mill (page 217). Keep in mind that not all home grain mills are equipped to do so, however, make sure yours does before using or purchasing. Even still, some grain mills are able to grind dried corn but not dried hominy, which is slightly larger and may have trouble getting through the small mouth of the mill. If that's the case, spread a flour sack towel onto a table and place a small pile of hominy in the center. Fold the edges of the towel over the top of the corn, and use a rolling pin to pound the corn into smaller pieces. Check the corn for any remaining whole pieces and continue to pound until every piece is cracked. Once cracked, the mill should accept the corn with ease. Remember, hominy grits (equivalent to polenta) are *coarsely ground* dried hominy—perfect in our Hominy Pie (page 144)—and masa harina (equivalent to corn flour) is *finely ground* dried hominy, which is used to make tortillas, tamales, and more.

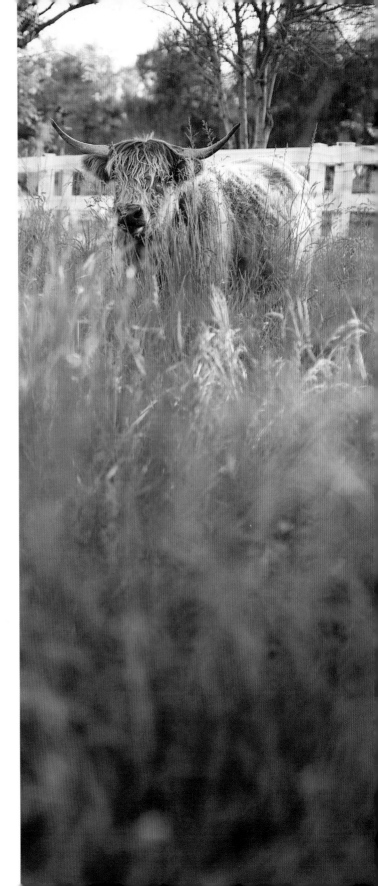

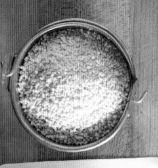

HONEY
GRANULES

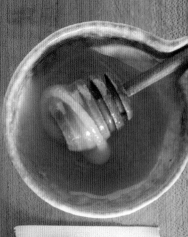

RAW
HONEY

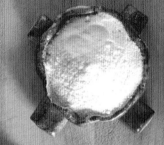

POWDERED
HONEY GRANULES

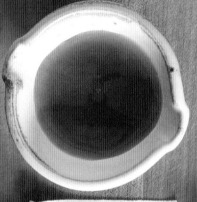

MAPLE
SYRUP

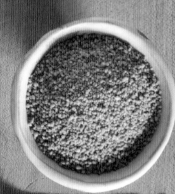

SUCANAT

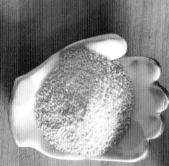

MAPLE
CRYSTALS

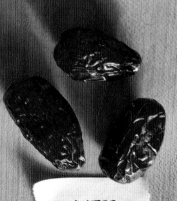

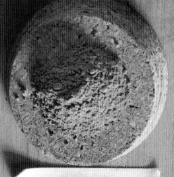

GREEN
STEVIA

DATES

CHAPTER 5

NATURAL SWEETENERS

ENDING OUR SUGAR ADDICTION

Our entire family was born with one gigantic sweet tooth. Every last one of us has found ultimate bliss in a warm cookie—then again, who hasn't?

But over the years, we began to discover the downfalls of white sugar: low energy, frequent colds, moodiness, and even more cravings. Desperate for a fix (and on our way to Traditional Foods), we experimented with more natural sweeteners, and low and behold, we felt better. But it wasn't until we relegated sweets—even natural ones—to "treat" status that we really noticed a difference. What does that mean? Well for one, the candy bowl gets removed from its permanent post on the counter. Dessert is more of a *no* than a *yes*, and sodas are an absolute rarity. We feel that kids should be rewarded with hugs and stickers over candy and we also feel, based on the personal experience of our own bodies, that radiant health cannot be achieved without sugar becoming a *condiment* and not an *entrée*.

> "Radiant health cannot be achieved without sugar becoming a *condiment* and not an *entrée.*"

All of this might sound depressing If you're a sugar addict, but we have an amazingly effective secret for you: If the amount of healthy fats in a diet goes up, sugar cravings go down. Fats make you feel fuller and more satiated, and keep your blood sugar levels balanced. As a result, your cravings go down—way down—and are replaced with more wholesome desires.

OUR FAVORITE NATURAL SWEETENERS

The next segment is a breakdown of the natural sweeteners commonly used in a Traditional Foods diet (and in this cookbook), most of which can be found at your local health food store (but visit the Resources section on page 216 if you're having any trouble sourcing). **Organic** is recommended for all.

And remember, these sweeteners, with the exception of powdered green stevia, should still be regarded as an *occasional* treat and used in moderation.

POWDERED HONEY GRANULES: THE POWDERED SUGAR SUBSTITUTE

Powdered honey granules are honey granules broken down to reach a texture similar to that of refined powdered sugar. One cup of honey granules yields 1 cup (120 g) of powdered honey granules.

TO MAKE: Measure the desired amount into the bowl of a blender. Cover and blend on high speed. Stop every 10 seconds to redistribute the granules. Continue blending until the granules are powdered, but avoid over-blending. The motor of the blender can melt the granules. Store in an airtight glass container in a cool pantry for several months. Warm temperatures may cause the powder to harden over time. Simply reprocess in the blender.

SUCANAT: *SU*-gar *CA*-ne *NAT*-ural

Sucanat is pure, dried sugar cane juice. Unlike common white sugar, Sucanat is unrefined and therefore contains the molasses mineral content typically lost in the refining process, resulting in a rustic color and deep flavor. Aesthetically, Sucanat's closest relative is brown sugar, for which a 1:1 substitution is commonplace; however, Sucanat is more granular, less moist, and more nutritious (brown sugar is typically common white sugar with just a bit of molasses added back). Sucanat is featured in our Chips Off the Old Block (page 138) and Sweet Ham Loaf (page 195).

RAW HONEY: NATURE'S LIQUID SWEETENER

Most store-bought honey is pasteurized, meaning it has been heated and strained to obtain a clear product that is easier to pour. Unfortunately, during this pasteurization process, many of the beneficial bacteria and enzymes, which help our bodies break down the sweetener, are destroyed. Unpasteurized or raw honey, on the other hand, still contains these valuable properties.

Raw honey can be thick and pastelike, but not always. Although a thick raw honey can be used in equal measure for a pourable raw variety, sourcing the latter combines ease of use with healthy benefits. And though the heat of recipe preparation negates many of these positive properties, we still recommend purchasing raw honey for cooking and baking, as we find the overall quality of the honey to be more consistent, and we prefer supporting farmers who choose less refinement in their practices. That said, even pasteurized honey is still a better choice than white sugar.

Raw honey substitutes 1:1 for liquid sweeteners. We feature it in our Roasted Shrimp Salsa (page 70), and Red Rice Salad with Cumin Dressing (page 109).

HONEY GRANULES: THE WHITE SUGAR SUBSTITUTE

Honey granules are a unique sweetener made from a combination of unrefined sugar cane juice (Sucanat) and honey, which is added to lighten the color and texture of the final product. Honey granules are the most accurate 1:1 natural sweetener swap for white sugar. The color of the final product will be earthier, resulting in a cream/eggshell color over a pure white. Honey granules are featured in our Sweet Onion Dressing (page 110) and E-Anne's Shortcakes (page 204).

REAL MAPLE SYRUP: CONTAINS ONLY ONE INGREDIENT

Real maple syrup comes from a maple tree; fake maple syrup is colored sugar water. Look at the ingredients carefully before buying—if they include only maple syrup, you've found the mother ship! The flavor will be richly sweet and full. This lovely natural sweetener comes in varying grades; Grade A is considered "premier" because of color and clarity and is perfect for drizzling over a warm sourdough pancake, while Grade B is usually cloudier and darker in color and is suggested for cooking and baking. Real maple syrup substitutes 1:1 for any liquid sweetener and is featured in both our Sticky Chicken (page 130) and Sprouted Apple Butter Dots (page 199).

MAPLE SUGAR: DEHYDRATED MAPLE SYRUP

Maple sugar (or crystals) is simply dehydrated maple syrup, and what a treat it is! The sugar can be substituted 1:1 for white sugar, but keep in mind it does add maple flavor and an extra soft fluffiness to the final texture of baked goods, which can be quite nice in the case of cookies and cakes. The sugar can also be pricey, so use it conservatively. Maple sugar is featured in Sourdough Bread Pudding with Raisins (page 190) and our Maple Walnut Cake with Cream Cheese Frosting (page 203).

POWDERED GREEN STEVIA: A SWEET PLANT WITHOUT THE "CRASH"

Stevia is an herb native to South America, where its natural green leaves are traditionally steeped in tea to impart a pleasantly sweet taste. The leaves can also be dried and crushed into a fine green powder. Many people who are intolerant of all sweeteners, even natural ones, enjoy powdered green stevia with no side effects.

An additional refinement process can turn the green powder to white, but we feel it also imparts a bitter aftertaste, reminiscent of artificial sweeteners, and refinement is something we work hard to avoid. We also find the white version to be much stronger, so we stick to the most natural version. Due to its natural green color, however, powdered stevia is best used in a recipe where the green color blends well into the deeper hue of other ingredients, such as in our Chester Cookies (page 196).

Powdered green stevia is significantly stronger than white sugar; approximately 1 teaspoon (2.5 g) can replace ¼ cup (50 g) sugar. Stevia also works well in tandem with another sweetener. For example, 1 teaspoon (2.5 g) of powdered green stevia plus ¼ cup (80 g) raw honey results in a taste that is similar in strength and flavor to ½ cup (160 g) raw honey.

DATES: NATURE'S CANDY

Let's clarify: In saying "date," we are referring to the whole, dried fruit, not the chopped, sugar-coated dates that appeared in the 1980s to make fruitcakes at Christmas. Several varieties of whole, dried dates are available at the farmers' markets in California and other desert climates, but the king of all dates, the Medjool date, is available in most grocery stores and truly satisfies even the most persistent sweet tooth. Dates are featured in our lightly sweet and refreshing Lemon Vinaigrette (page 112) and the quick, satisfying snack Almond Boy (page 207).

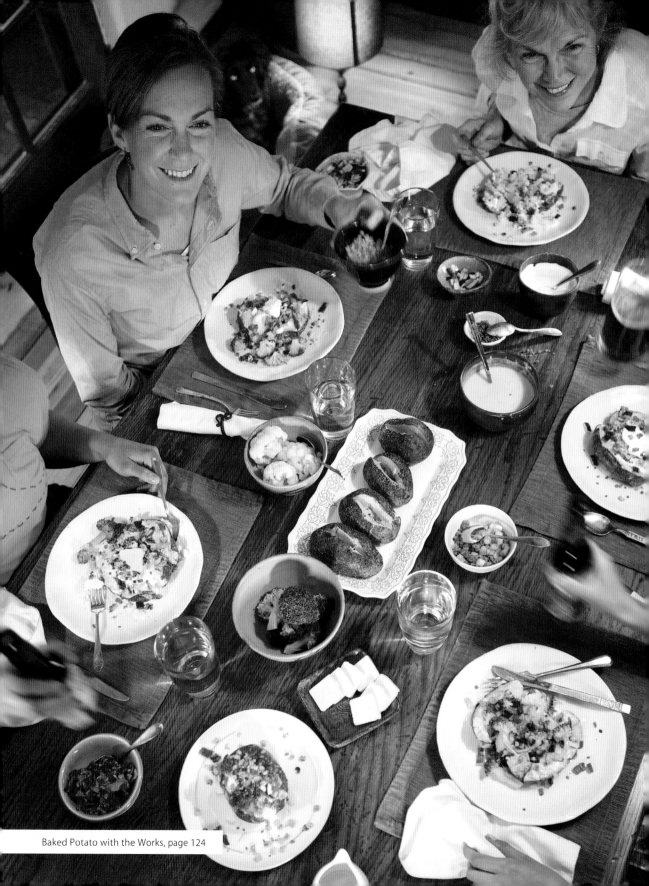

Baked Potato with the Works, page 124

PART 2

TRADITIONAL FOODS RECIPES

When you step into the kitchen and tie on that apron, you're more than a cook—you're an artist. Consider the stove your easel and the ingredients your paint. As these recipes were developed, you were forefront in our thoughts. Our efforts are complete when you succeed. That said, every artistic endeavor has a learning curve. Beginnings are rarely magical. But magic does happen when you just keep putting on that apron!

"Practice isn't the thing you do when you're good. It's the thing you do that *makes* you good."
—Malcolm Gladwell, *Outliers: The Story of Success*

AN INGREDIENT REMINDER

We've mentioned this in our introduction, but it bears repeating here: to avoid clutter, we omit certain descriptive words in the ingredient lists of the recipes. For example:

- Organic is not placed before, well, *everything*! But we certainly recommend it be so.
- We recommend all meat and eggs be pastured, also known as grass-fed (page 35).
- All seafood is wild with sustainable certification, such as MSC certification.
- All butter used in the creation of the recipes was pastured and unsalted.
- We recommend all other dairy—including milk, cream, and cheese—be sourced as grass-fed, whole/full-fat and possibly raw for uncooked applications (page 37).
- We highly recommend a quality mineral-rich fine sea salt, rather than refined table salt.
- In our baking recipes, we rely on fresh-milled, sprouted flour, which creates very light, airy flour. Regular store-bought flour will not produce the same result.
- All vinegar is unfiltered.
- All honey is raw.
- All water is filtered.

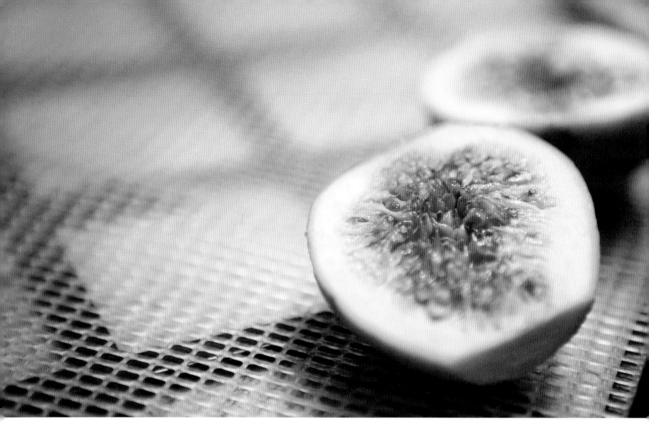

CHAPTER 6

FIRST BITES

LET'S BE HONEST—we don't make a whole lot of appetizers for a typical family dinner. These dishes are pulled out for company, a welcome nod for someone special. The last few minutes in an entertaining kitchen can be hectic. An appetizer acts like a shiny object, distracting guests from noticing any kitchen mishaps. One night, I actually returned a sheet pan to the oven with a potholder stuck on the bottom, but thanks to the Roasted Shrimp Salsa (page 70), our guests "barely" noticed the billowing smoke!

back to butter

One of the great things about having a big garden is having lots of culinary herbs. It may feel excessive to buy the four bunches of parsley to make tabbouleh, but not when it's plentiful in your garden! Typically made with bulgur wheat, this salad substitutes in quinoa, which allows our gluten-free friends to partake. I like serving it with cucumber rounds.

Quinoa Tabbouleh

3 cups (555 g) cooked quinoa (page 53)

¾ cup (109 g) dried currants

1 cup (180 g) seeded and diced tomato

3 cups (180 g) chopped fresh flat-leaf parsley (about 4 bunches)

¾ cup (75 g) diagonally sliced scallion, both white and green parts

⅓ cup (80 ml) lemon juice

⅓ cup (80 ml) extra-virgin olive oil

½ teaspoon garlic paste

1 teaspoon sea salt

½ teaspoon freshly cracked pepper

YIELD: 8 CUPS (1,800 G), OR 10 TO 12 SERVINGS

Combine the quinoa, currants, tomato, parsley, and scallion in a large-size bowl. With a fork, toss the ingredients to combine.

In a separate bowl, whisk the lemon juice, olive oil, garlic, sea salt, and pepper. Pour over the quinoa mixture and using your fork, toss again.

Chill for 2 hours, if desired, and serve.

RECIPE NOTES

• To seed a tomato, cut the tomato in half from top to bottom and scoop out the seeds and "gel" of the tomato with your finger or a spoon. It is not necessary to remove the more dense tomato "ribs." The tomato seeds are removed to avoid adding excess liquid to the salad.

• A food processor is a quick way to chop this amount of parsley. Remove the coarse parsley stems before chopping. The parsley should be dried thoroughly before chopping. A salad spinner makes this a breeze—or just pat dry with a kitchen towel.

• To make garlic paste: Mince the garlic on a cutting board. Once minced, sprinkle a pinch of coarse sea salt over the top. Chop some more. Then, using the flat side of a knife, carefully press down firmly on the garlic and drag the knife along the cutting board and through the garlic. Pile the garlic again and repeat until it forms a paste.

If you only grow one thing, grow a tomato plant. Upon your first taste of a homegrown, sun-ripened tomato, you'll understand why. And if you grow little grape tomatoes, this recipe is a must. Serve with Multi-Seed Crackers (page 76) for a great way to start off a cookout.

Roasted Shrimp Salsa

FOR SHRIMP:

½ pound (225 g) 16/20 count shrimp, peeled, deveined, and tails removed

1 tablespoon (14 g) coconut oil

¼ teaspoon ground coriander

½ teaspoon sea salt

½ teaspoon freshly cracked pepper

FOR SALSA:

1 cup (180 g) halved grape tomatoes

¼ cup (38 g) small diced yellow pepper

¼ cup (30 g) peeled, seeded, and small diced cucumber

1 tablespoon (9 g) minced jalapeño

¼ cup (40 g) minced red onion

1 tablespoon (4 g) chopped fresh flat-leaf parsley

2 tablespoons (30 ml) fresh lime juice

2 tablespoons (30 ml) extra-virgin olive oil

2 teaspoons raw honey (page 64)

1 teaspoon garlic paste (see Note, page 69)

¼ teaspoon ground coriander

1 teaspoon sea salt

½ teaspoon freshly cracked pepper

1 cup (146 g) medium diced avocado

TO MAKE THE SHRIMP: Preheat the oven to 400ºF (200ºC, or gas mark 6). Rinse the shrimp and dry thoroughly with a paper towel.

Add the coconut oil to a small-size sheet tray (although any size will do). If the coconut oil is solidified, place the tray in the oven as it preheats for 2 minutes, to melt the oil.

To the pan, add the shrimp, coriander, sea salt, and pepper. Toss well with a spatula and bake for 7 minutes. Remove from the heat and re-toss the shrimp. Transfer to a plate to cool.

TO MAKE THE SALSA: In a medium-size bowl, combine the tomatoes, yellow pepper, cucumber, jalapeño, red onion, and parsley. Set aside. In a small-size bowl, combine the lime juice, olive oil, honey, garlic, coriander, salt, and pepper. Whisk to combine. Pour the dressing over the tomato mixture. Toss gently with a spatula to combine.

Dice the cooled shrimp into ½-inch (1.3 cm) pieces. If serving immediately, add the shrimp and avocado to the tomato mixture. Toss gently with a spatula to combine and serve.

If not serving immediately, toss the shrimp with the tomato mixture and chill. Right before serving, add the avocado and serve.

YIELD: 6 TO 8 SERVINGS, OR 3 CUPS (780 G)

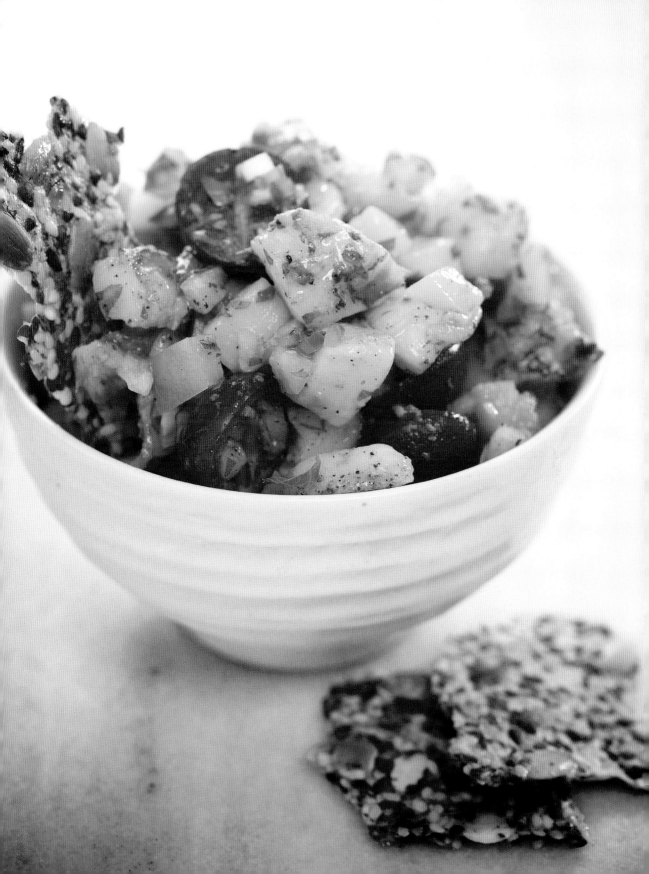

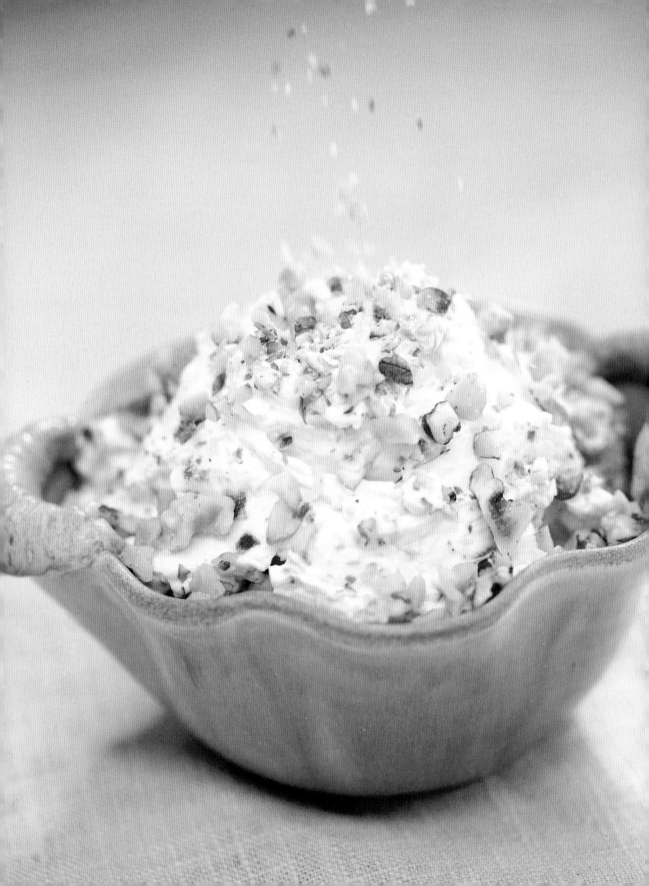

Do you remember cream cheese balls that were rolled in walnuts and served at most holiday gatherings? Here's a wholesome take on that classic appetizer. Here, we use our homemade tangy cream cheese and creamy mayonnaise. Goodbye additives, hello flavor!

Cultured Cream Cheese Olive Dip

8 ounces (225 g) Yogurt Cream Cheese (page 40)

2 tablespoons (28 g) Simply Mayonnaise (page 178)

1 teaspoon fish sauce (page 217)

2 tablespoons (12 g) minced black olives

2 tablespoons (12 g) minced green olives

1 tablespoon (10 g) minced sweet onion

1 tablespoon (4 g) chopped fresh flat-leaf parsley

½ cup (60 g) finely grated white Cheddar cheese

¼ cup (28 g) finely chopped crunchy walnuts (page 49)

YIELD: 8 SERVINGS, OR 1⅓ CUPS (306 G)

In a medium-size bowl, combine the cream cheese, mayonnaise, fish sauce, black olives, green olives, onion, and parsley. Combine with a hand mixer. Fold in the cheese with a spatula until thoroughly combined.

Spread the dip into a small-size ceramic dish fitted with its own lid, which is helpful for storage while chilling. Chill for at least 1 hour before serving.

Coat the top of the dip thoroughly with chopped walnuts. Serve cold with crackers, sliced vegetables, or sliced apples.

RECIPE NOTE

To finely grate white Cheddar cheese, it is necessary to use a microplane grater, which is a very convenient kitchen tool that's also great for zesting citrus and grating Parmesan.

After one taste of this hummus, you may permanently retire the store-bought variety. Homemade is cheaper, fluffier, and it's easier! It allows endless flavor options. Green Olive and Sun-Dried Tomato are shared below, but feel free to create your own!

Homemade Hummus
Traditional, Green Olive, or Sun-Dried Tomato

FOR TRADITIONAL HUMMUS:

1 clove garlic, peeled

⅓ cup (80 g) tahini

¼ cup (60 ml) freshly squeezed lemon juice

½ cup (120 ml) water

½ teaspoon sea salt

⅛ teaspoon cayenne pepper

3 cups (720 g) cooked chickpeas (page 52)

FOR GREEN OLIVE HUMMUS:

¾ cup (75 g) pitted green olives

1 recipe Traditional Hummus

FOR SUN-DRIED TOMATO HUMMUS:

½ cup (27 g) sun-dried tomatoes (*not* packed in oil)

1 cup (235 ml) hot water

1 recipe Traditional Hummus, made with tomato soaking liquid instead of water

FOR GARNISH:

Extra-virgin olive oil

TO MAKE THE TRADITIONAL HUMMUS: Using a food processor, chop the garlic until minced. Add the tahini, lemon juice, water, sea salt, and cayenne. Process until smooth and well combined.

Add the cooked and drained chickpeas and process again, scraping down the sides of the bowl as necessary. Once blended, process for 1 additional minute. The extra processing gives the hummus a fluffy texture. Serve immediately or chill.

TO MAKE THE GREEN OLIVE HUMMUS: Add the green olives to the bowl of the food processor. Process for 5 seconds until just chopped. Using a spatula, scrape the olives into a small-size bowl. Complete the traditional recipe above, then add the olives back into the bowl and pulse to combine.

TO MAKE THE SUN-DRIED TOMATO HUMMUS: Soak the sun-dried tomatoes in the hot water for 10 minutes. Drain and reserve ½ cup (120 ml) of the soaking liquid. Add the sun-dried tomatoes to the bowl of the food processor. Process for 30 seconds or until just chopped. Using a spatula, scrape the tomatoes into a small-size bowl. Proceed with the traditional recipe above, but substitute the soaking liquid for the water. Add the sun-dried tomatoes back into the bowl and pulse to combine.

TO SERVE: Drizzle with extra-virgin olive oil and serve with sliced vegetables or seed crackers.

YIELD: 3 CUPS (675 G)

The French know how to use butter, as this pâté recipe wonderfully highlights. If you've never made or tried one before, a pâté is a spread made by combining a cooked meat with a fat. In this case, we feature two of the most nutrient dense foods available—butter and organ meat. The result is an amazingly smooth and tasty delight that is perfect spread on our Multi-Seed Crackers (page 76). See for yourself how delicious liver can be!

Chicken Liver Pâté

1 pound (454 g) chicken liver, washed and connective tissue removed

1 thick (½-inch, or 12 mm) slice sweet onion

4 large cloves peeled garlic, whole

8 tablespoons (112 g) butter, at room temperature, cut into 8 chunks

¾ cup (75 g) Parmesan

¾ teaspoon sea salt

¼ teaspoon black pepper

YIELD: 2½ CUPS, OR 8 TO 10 SERVINGS

Place liver in a large saucepan. Add the onion and garlic and cover completely with water. Bring to a boil, cover, and simmer gently for 5 minutes, turning down heat as required. Remove from heat and let stand, covered, for 10 minutes.

Drain liver mixture well. Roughly cut onion into large chunks, then place the drained liver, cut onion, and garlic into the bowl of the food processor. Process for 25 seconds, or until the mixture is smooth.

With motor running, add butter, one tablespoon (14 g) at a time, through the mouth of the processor. Allow each piece to fully incorporate into the warm liver before adding the next.

Once all the butter has been incorporated, remove lid and add Parmesan, then season with salt and pepper. Process the mixture for about 10 additional seconds to combine.

Transfer mixture to a 9-inch (23 cm) tart dish or several individual ramekins, as desired. Refrigerate for 1 to 2 hours, uncovered, before serving. Once thoroughly chilled, serve with crackers or fresh vegetables. Store leftovers in covered container in fridge.

If you don't own a dehydrator (page 51), this recipe may sound a bit complicated and intimidating. But once you have one, you will take to this recipe with ease. The technique is basic, and the yield is high, making the effort worth the result. You can keep the crackers at room temperature for a week, or store in the freezer for several months. This recipe features golden flaxseed, though traditional brown flaxseed is also suitable if you can't locate the lighter variety. Note that there is a minimum of 12 hours of advance prep time.

Multi-Seed Crackers

2 cups (288 g) raw golden flaxseed

2 cups (288 g) raw hulled sesame seeds

2 cups (288 g) raw hulled pumpkin seeds

2 tablespoons (36 g) sea salt, plus more to taste, divided

½ cup (80 g) diced shallot (about 2 medium)

1 tablespoon (6 g) minced garlic

¼ teaspoon cayenne pepper

YIELD: 1-GALLON (3.7 L) SIZE CONTAINER OF CRACKERS

In a medium-size ceramic or glass bowl, combine the flaxseed with 4 cups (940 ml) water. Stir, cover, and set aside for 12 hours. In a larger ceramic or glass bowl, combine the sesame seeds, pumpkin seeds, 1 tablespoon (18 g) of the sea salt, and enough water to cover by 2 inches (5 cm). Stir, cover, and set aside to soak for 12 hours.

After soaking, drain and rinse the pumpkin and sesame seeds in a mesh strainer. Set aside. Do *not* rinse the flaxseed.

Once soaked, the flaxseed will be gelatinous and have absorbed most of the liquid. The gelatinous nature of soaked flax is needed to bind the cracker. To the flaxseed, add the shallot, garlic, remaining 1 tablespoon (18 g) sea salt, and cayenne pepper. Stir with a wooden spoon to combine.

Using a food processor, grind the flax mixture in two batches, 1 minute per batch. Most seeds will be broken down, but some will remain whole. Into a large-size bowl, recombine both batches and add the pumpkin seeds and sesame seeds. Using a spatula, fold the mixture together until thoroughly combined.

Line 5 dehydrator trays with nonstick sheets (such as those used for fruit leather). Spread about 2 cups (320 g) of batter evenly onto each tray using an offset or rubber spatula. Spread to a ¼-inch (6 mm) thickness. Sprinkle with sea salt and dehydrate at 150ºF (66ºC) for 12 hours.

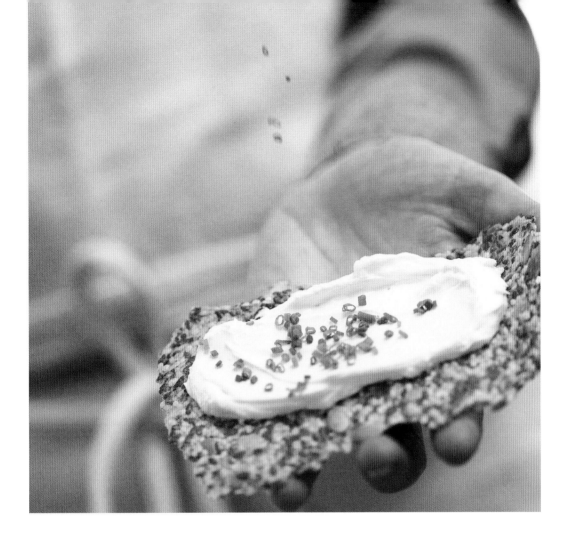

After 12 hours, remove and flip the crackers. Do this by laying the cracker sheet on an even surface and placing a mesh dehydrator liner on top. Invert the tray so it's face down on top of the mesh liner. Carefully peel the top nonstick sheet from the cracker and return the flipped cracker, now on the mesh liner, to the dehydrator for another 6 hours at 150°F (66ºC) to dry completely.

After 6 hours, turn off the heat, open the dehydrator, and allow the crackers to cool completely. Remove the crackers, break into large-size pieces, and store in an airtight container at room temperature for 1 week or transfer to a freezer for several months.

RECIPE NOTE

Try spreading one of these crackers with grass-fed butter and a spoonful of salty wild salmon roe (page 216), a delicious and nutrient-dense snack! Salmon roe was considered a sacred food among traditional cultures.

first bites

Having grown up in Atlanta, Georgia, I associate summer with sweet Vidalia onions, truly nature's candy. The onions get their name from Vidalia, Georgia, where the low-sulfur soil gives them their uniquely sweet taste, perfect for this dip. If you can't find Vidalia, substitute some other sweet variety, such as a Maui or Walla Walla.

Hot Onion Dip

Inspired by Jean Desvernine

¾ cup (175 g) Simply Mayonnaise (page 178)

1 teaspoon minced garlic

1 teaspoon hot sauce

1 teaspoon minced horseradish

2 cups (320 g) small diced Vidalia onion

1½ cups (165 g) grated Swiss cheese

YIELD: 4 TO 6 SERVINGS, OR 2½ CUPS (565 G)

Preheat the oven to 350ºF (180ºC, or gas mark 4). Have ready a 9-inch (23 cm) pie pan or an 8 x 8-inch (20 x 20 cm) glass baking dish (no need to grease). In a medium-size bowl, combine the mayonnaise, garlic, hot sauce, and horseradish. Add the onion and stir until fully incorporated. Add the Swiss cheese and stir again.

Pour the mixture into the dish and level with a spatula. Bake for 25 to 30 minutes, until the cheese is melted and the edges have turned golden brown.

Cool for 5 minutes and serve warm with crackers or veggies.

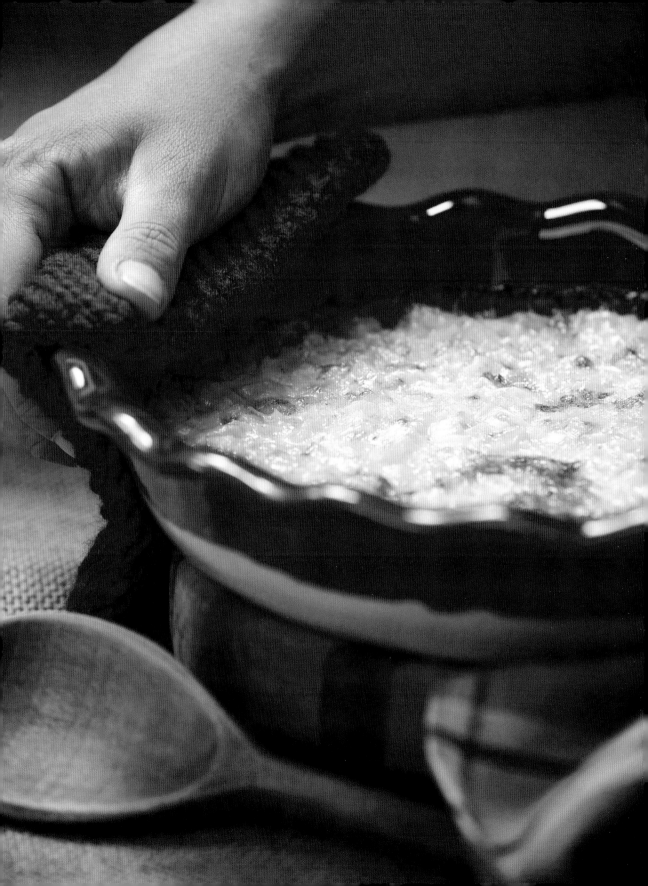

Living on a farm with acres of avocado trees, I've had my fair share of guacamole. Although our livestock assistant, Flavio, still makes the best guacamole I know, my roasted corn version has its own fan following. Keep in mind that the lemon juice and avocado are combined in the very first step of the guacamole, because the acid prevents the avocado from turning brown. This attention to detail will preserve the beautiful green color of the dip.

Roasted Corn Guacamole

1 tablespoon (14 g) butter

½ cup (75 g) corn

⅛ plus ¼ teaspoon sea salt, divided

⅛ plus ¼ teaspoon pepper, divided

2 avocados

4 teaspoons (20 ml) fresh lemon juice

⅓ cup (60 g) seeded and small diced tomato

¼ cup (40 g) finely diced red onion

1 teaspoon minced garlic

YIELD: 1½ CUPS (338 G)

Preheat the oven to 350ºF (180ºC, or gas mark 4). While the oven is preheating, put the butter on a small-size baking tray and place in the oven for 2 to 4 minutes to melt.

Once the butter is melted, remove the tray and place the corn on it. Sprinkle with ⅛ teaspoon of the sea salt and ⅛ teaspoon of the pepper and toss with a spatula to combine. Roast for 25 minutes, tossing once halfway through, until the corn is browned. Set aside to cool while prepping the remaining ingredients.

Peel and dice the avocados and combine in a small-size bowl with the lemon juice. Mash with a fork or potato masher, leaving the mixture slightly chunky. Add the tomatoes, red onion, garlic, remaining ¼ teaspoon sea salt, and remaining ¼ teaspoon pepper. Toss with a fork to combine, then fold in the roasted and cooled corn. Serve immediately.

RECIPE NOTES

• Fresh corn cut from the cob will supply the most flavor, but frozen corn may be substituted. If corn is frozen, it is best not to thaw before using.

• Guacamole oxidizes and turns brown quickly. If you need to store it, place the dip in a glass container and press a piece of plastic wrap down onto the top surface of the dip; the entire surface of the dip should be touching the plastic. Put the lid on top and refrigerate.

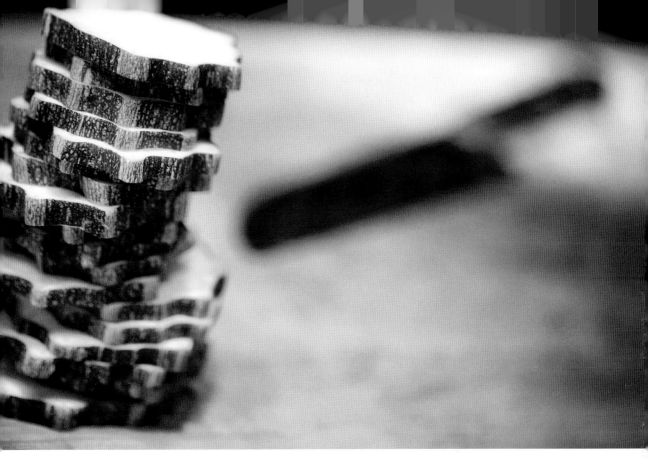

CHAPTER 7

SOUP'S ON

ON A FARM, death and life rest a nose's distance away from a naked eye. A baby lamb fills every acre with exuberant joy, whereas a stillborn aches the heart, no matter how many times it's experienced. My first slaughter was a rooster. We had too many, and on a farm, hard decisions are inevitable. I didn't know what to expect, but I certainly didn't anticipate the peace, quiet, and respect that permeated the surroundings. An animal that lives an appropriate life, with space, clean water, and proper food, one chosen for death in order to nourish another body, dies a peaceful death—and becomes the most amazing chicken soup that's ever been eaten.

Slow-cooked homemade stocks are a cook's key to a strong and robust family! The 24-hour cook time pulls more gelatin and nutrients from the bones, serving as nature's protection from osteoporosis and weak joints. Any combination of chicken pieces will work. Backs and wings, left over from breaking down a whole chicken or purchased from your butcher, serve as inexpensive and effective stock meat. And this may sound odd, but chicken feet add tons of joint-protecting gelatin to the stock, which can actually make the stock "gel" in the fridge. Sip a warm cup of homemade stock first thing in the morning with nothing but a pinch of sea salt. My husband and I do this all the time and it makes for a great start to the day.

Nourishing Chicken Stock

5 quarts (4.5 L) cold water

2 tablespoons (30 ml) apple cider vinegar

2 pounds (908 g) bone-in chicken, any cut or size

4 chicken feet, optional

2 cups (240 g) carrots cut into 2-inch (5 cm) pieces

3 cups (300 g) celery cut into 2-inch (5 cm) pieces, leaves left on

2 fresh or dried bay leaves

10 whole black peppercorns

1 large onion, peeled and quartered

2 cloves garlic, whole and unpeeled

8 sprigs parsley

YIELD: ABOUT 4 QUARTS (3.6 L)

In a large-size pot, combine the cold water, apple cider vinegar, chicken, and chicken feet, if using. Allow the chicken to soak in the vinegar water for 1 hour, drawing additional calcium from the bones.

Bring the water to a boil over high heat, uncovered. A foamy scum may develop on the surface of the stock once a rolling boil is reached. Skim this and discard. The foam is natural coagulated lipoprotein. It's not harmful but it isn't pretty either and may cloud the stock. Add the remaining ingredients, except the parsley, to the pot (this will be added at the very end of cooking).

Cover and reduce the heat to low, maintaining a gentle simmer. It's important to keep the pot covered, as this allows the stock to bubble away for hours without fear of the liquid evaporating. Simmer for anywhere from 12 to 24 hours, depending on how much time you have, adjusting the heat up or down as needed. A long cooking time allows more digestion-enhancing gelatin to be released from the bones into the stock and enhances its flavor. If you have time for a 24-hour stock, occasionally check the stock and, if necessary, add more water to ensure the meat is covered.

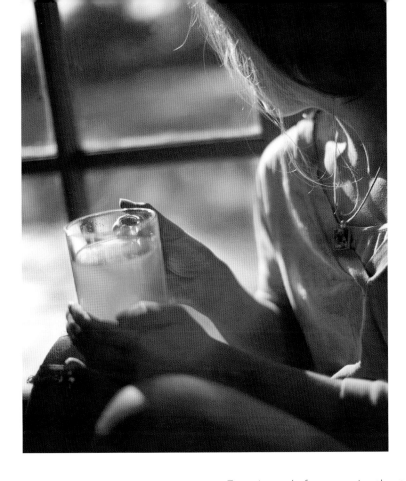

Ten minutes before removing the stock from the heat, add the parsley. Once done, remove from the heat and cool, uncovered, for 10 minutes. Strain the stock using a chinois (see Note) or large-size strainer. Stock may be used immediately. However, when fully cooled in the refrigerator, any fat will rise to the surface and congeal. Use a slotted spoon to carefully scoop off the fat and set aside for reuse (it's great for sautéing vegetables or frying eggs). This step allows the cook to control the amount of fat in the final dish.

RECIPE NOTE

A chinois is the Rolls Royce of kitchen strainers. Its long handle and fine mesh make straining something such as bone broth simple and efficient. When the stock is passed through the chinois only one time, it becomes clear and perfectly strained. Because a common kitchen strainer has much larger holes than a chinois, many passes and usually cheesecloth are required to reach a comparable result.

Both ox tails and short ribs are excellent choices for bone-in cuts of meat. Many grocery stores already have knuckle and marrowbones packaged in the freezer section for purchase. If not, ask a favorite butcher to save them for you. Better yet, seek out grass-fed beef from a local farmers' market; it will be a much less expensive option.

Nourishing Beef Stock

6 quarts (5.4 L) cold water

2 pounds (908 g) beef bone marrow and/or knuckle bones

2 tablespoons (30 ml) apple cider vinegar

2 pounds (908 g) bone-in cuts of meat

1 teaspoon sea salt

1 teaspoon freshly cracked black pepper

3 cups (360 g) carrots cut into 2-inch (5 cm) pieces

3 cups (300 g) celery cut into 2-inch (5 cm) pieces, leaves left on

2 fresh or dried bay leaves

10 whole black peppercorns

1 large onion, peeled and quartered

2 cloves garlic, whole and unpeeled

8 sprigs parsley

YIELD: ABOUT 4 QUARTS (3.8 L)

Preheat the oven to 400ºF (200ºC, or gas mark 6). In a 12-quart (11 L) stockpot, combine the water, bone marrow, and apple cider vinegar. Allow the bones to soak in the solution for 1 hour, to draw out calcium from the bones.

Reserving the soaking solution in the stockpot, place the meaty beef bones on a sheet pan. Sprinkle evenly with sea salt and pepper. Roast in the oven for 40 to 60 minutes to produce a crispy, brown exterior, which will ultimately help flavor the stock. Note that some cuts, such as oxtails, require less cooking time.

Once the bones brown, remove them from the oven. Using tongs, add them back to the stockpot. Bring the water to a boil over high heat, uncovered. A foamy scum may develop on the surface of the stock once a rolling boil is reached. If you like you can skim this and discard. The foam is natural coagulated lipoprotein. It's not harmful but it isn't pretty either and may cloud the stock.

Add the remaining ingredients, except the parsley, to the pot (this will be added at the very end of cooking), cover and reduce the heat to low, maintaining a gentle simmer. It's important to keep the stockpot covered, as this allows the stock to bubble away for hours without fear of the liquid evaporating. Simmer for anywhere from 12 to 24 hours, depending on how much time you have, adjusting the heat up or down as

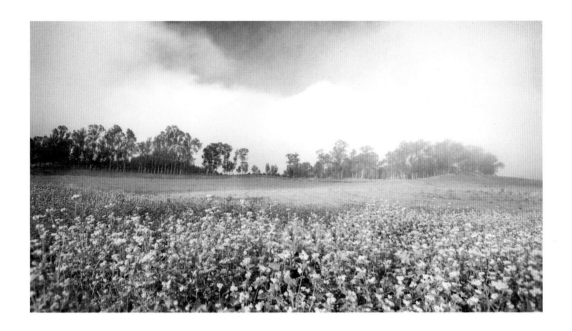

needed. A long cooking time allows more digestion-enhancing gelatin to be released from the bones into the stock and enhances its flavor. If you have time for the 24-hour stock, occasionally check to ensure the meat is covered with liquid, adding more water as needed.

Ten minutes before removing the stock from the heat, add the parsley. Once done, remove from the heat and cool uncovered for 10 minutes. Using a pair of tongs, remove large bones and discard. Strain the stock with a chinois (page 83) or large strainer. The stock may be used immediately. However, when fully cooled in the refrigerator, any fat will rise to the surface and congeal. Use a slotted spoon to carefully scoop off the fat and set aside for reuse (it's great for sautéing vegetables or frying eggs). This step allows the cook to control the amount of fat in the final dish.

RECIPE NOTE

Store stock in a glass container in the fridge for up to a week, or stock may also be pressure canned to remain shelf-stable for up to a year. Stocks may be stored in the freezer for several months. To freeze, add stock to a 1-quart (1 L) glass Mason jar, making sure to allow 3 inches (7.5 cm) of room in the jar for the liquid to expand in the freezer. Resist boiling the jar in a pot of water to thaw; the glass jar can break. Instead, defrost on the counter, in the fridge, or in a pinch, in a bowl of warm water.

This soup originated as a recipe for a pilot TV show my husband and I created called *Farm to Table*. The show never made it off the ground, but the recipe has become a staple in our kitchen. The idea of "stuffing" soup comes from a wonderful market in Baltimore, Maryland, called Atwater's. Ned Atwater always serves the customers seated at the stools of his soup bar with something special scooped into the middle of their piping hot soup.

Zucchini Soup with Corn & Pancetta Stuffing

FOR SOUP:

1 tablespoon (14 g) coconut oil

2 cups (320 g) medium diced yellow onion

6 cups (720 g) medium diced zucchini (about 5 medium)

4 cups (940 ml) homemade chicken stock (page 82)

2 teaspoons (12 g) sea salt, plus more to taste

½ teaspoon pepper, plus more to taste

FOR STUFFING:

2 ounces (56 g) thinly sliced pancetta, diced into ½-inch (1.3 cm) pieces

½ pound (225 g) mild or hot uncooked, casing-free Italian chicken or turkey sausage

2 cups (300 g) fresh corn cut off the cob (about 2 ears)

Sprouts, for garnish

TO MAKE THE SOUP: In a medium-size pot over medium heat, melt the coconut oil until glistening. Add the onion and sauté for 5 minutes, stirring occasionally, until softened. Add the zucchini, chicken stock, sea salt, and pepper. Bring to a boil, then reduce the heat to maintain a rolling simmer. Cover and cook for 15 minutes, until softened.

Remove from the heat and allow the soup to cool for 5 minutes. Purée the mixture using an immersion blender or in a regular blender. Season with sea salt and pepper, if necessary.

TO MAKE THE STUFFING: In a large sauté pan over medium heat, add the pancetta and cook until crispy, stirring occasionally, about 5 minutes. Transfer pancetta to a paper towel–lined plate.

Add the sausage to the pan and break apart using a wooden spoon or potato masher. Cook for 5 minutes, until the meat is cooked through and lightly browned. Turn off the heat and add the pancetta back to the pan. Stir to combine. Fold in the fresh corn until fully combined.

To serve, ladle into soup bowls and place a large spoonful of the stuffing into the center of each bowl. Garnish with sprouts and serve warm.

YIELD: 4 SERVINGS

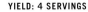

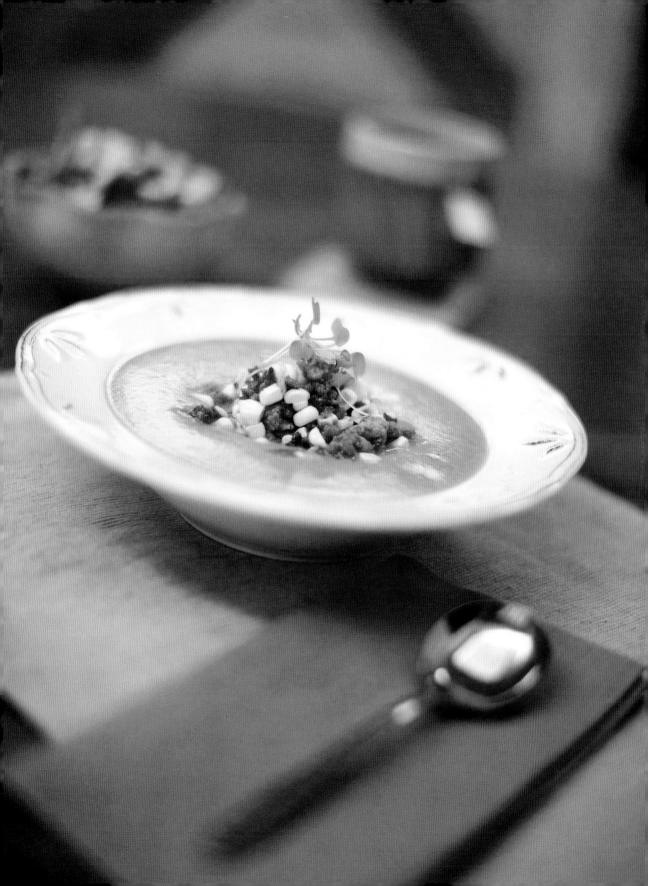

This soup is a great example of how little effort a good soup takes when started with an excellent homemade stock. If you don't own an immersion blender, a regular blender will bring the same result. Broccoli, cauliflower, or asparagus may be chosen as the main ingredient, allowing the same basic recipe to be taken in three completely different directions. I've been known to spend the whole day eating only this soup to give my digestive system a welcomed break.

Simple Puréed Soup
Broccoli, Cauliflower, or Asparagus

1 tablespoon (14 g) butter

1 cup (160 g) diced yellow onion

1 tablespoon (10 g) minced garlic

5 cups (500 g) cut-up broccoli, cauliflower, or asparagus

4 cups (940 ml) homemade chicken stock (page 82)

½ teaspoon crushed red pepper flakes

2½ teaspoons (15 g) sea salt

½ teaspoon freshly cracked pepper

YIELD: 6 SERVINGS

In a medium-size pot over medium heat, melt the butter until it begins to foam. Add the onion and sauté for 5 minutes, until softened. Add the garlic and sauté for 1 minute, until fragrant. Add chosen vegetable (broccoli, cauliflower, or asparagus), chicken stock, red pepper flakes, sea salt, and pepper. Bring to a boil. Cover and lower the heat to medium; cook for 10 minutes, maintaining a rolling simmer.

Remove from the heat. Uncover and cool for 5 minutes. Purée in the pot if using an immersion blender, or in a regular blender, until the mixture is smooth. Return to the pan (if necessary) and keep covered on low heat until ready to serve.

RECIPE NOTES

• For Broccoli Soup: Both the florets and the stems of the broccoli may be used. Cut the florets off the stem and into bite-size pieces. Trim the tough bottom inch (2.5 cm) from the stem and using a vegetable peeler, peel the outer layer. Cut into 1-inch (2.5 cm) chunks.

• For Cauliflower Soup: Both the florets and the tender stems may be used.

• An immersion blender—also known as a handheld blender or purée stick—is an inexpensive kitchen tool that makes puréeing soups quick and mess-free! When using this tool, slightly tilt the pot to create a deep well of soup. Lower the stick into the well and process.

In general, my body behaves properly when my overall intake of grains stays low. Therefore, when I choose to eat them, I make sure to use unrefined grains that have been properly treated according to the wisdom of traditional cultures. Classic minestrone uses refined semolina pasta, which is replaced in this recipe with whole-grain rice that has been properly soaked and prepared. We don't miss the pasta one bit!

Minestrone with Brown Rice

FOR SOUP:

1 tablespoon (14 g) butter

1 cup (160 g) diced onion

¾ cup (98 g) diced carrot

2 teaspoons (6 g) minced garlic

5 cups (1175 ml) homemade chicken
   stock (page 82)

½ cup (85 g) cooked brown rice
   (page 54)

2 cans (14 ounces, or 392 g each)
   diced tomatoes, with juice

1 tablespoon (3 g) chopped fresh basil

1 tablespoon (4 g) chopped fresh
   oregano

2 teaspoons (1 g) fresh thyme

2½ teaspoons (15 g) sea salt

½ teaspoon freshly cracked pepper

1 cup (150 g) diced turnip (about
   1 medium)

1½ cups (225 g) cooked cannelloni
   beans, plus ½ cup (120 ml) cooking
   liquid (page 52)

4 cups (120 g) roughly chopped
   packed baby spinach

FOR GARNISH:

⅔ cup (65 g) grated Parmesan

Extra-virgin olive oil, for drizzling

Freshly cracked pepper

TO MAKE THE SOUP: In a large-size pot, melt the butter over medium heat. Add the onion and carrot and sauté, stirring occasionally, for 5 minutes, until slightly softened. Add the garlic and sauté for 1 minute, stirring constantly, until fragrant. Add the stock, rice, tomatoes, basil, oregano, thyme, sea salt, and pepper. Bring to a boil. Cover, reduce the heat to medium-low, and maintain a rolling simmer for 40 minutes, adjusting the heat as necessary. Uncover and add the turnip, beans, and bean cooking liquid. Re-cover and continue to maintain a rolling simmer for an additional 30 minutes.

Remove from the heat. Fold in the spinach until just wilted.

TO SERVE: Serve family-style with the Parmesan, olive oil, and pepper on the side.

YIELD: 6 SERVINGS

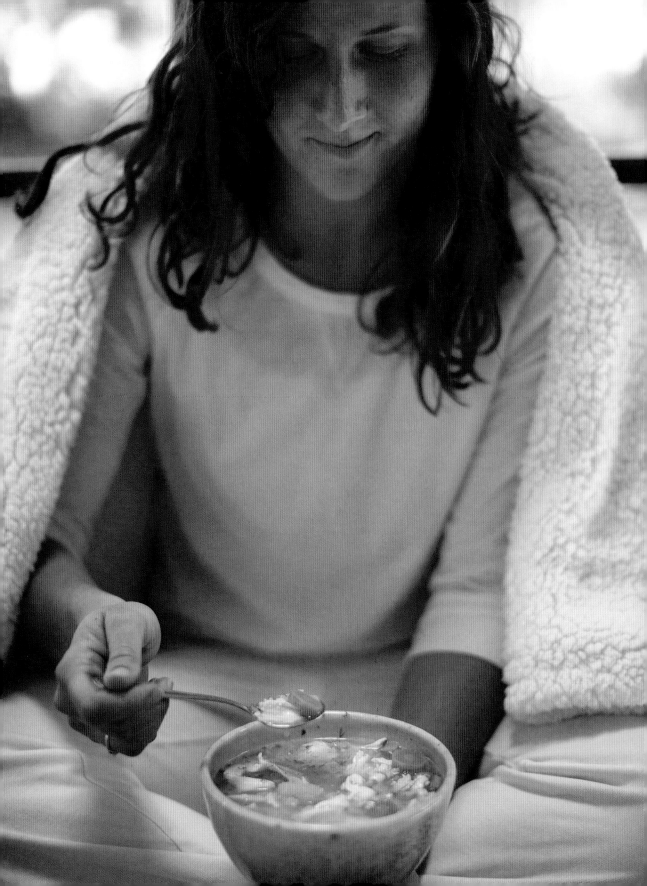

This wholesome and healing recipe is a staple in my house for cool winter evenings, but also for common colds. Brown rice replaces the more ordinary and less nutritious white rice, while the homemade chicken stock truly makes the dish. Dill is a classic chicken soup herb for good reason: It's delicious!

Chicken & Brown Rice Soup with Dill

2 tablespoons (28 g) butter

1 cup (160 g) finely diced yellow onion

1 cup (130 g) peeled and thinly sliced carrots, cut into half moons

1 cup (120 g) thinly sliced celery

1 tablespoon (10 g) minced garlic

8 cups (1880 ml) homemade chicken stock (page 82)

2 cups (280 g) cooked and shredded chicken breast (page 32)

2 cups (330 g) cooked brown rice (page 54)

2½ teaspoons (15 g) sea salt

½ teaspoon freshly cracked pepper

1 tablespoon (4 g) chopped fresh dill

In a large-size pot, melt the butter over medium heat. Add the onion, carrots, and celery. Sauté for 5 minutes, stirring occasionally, until the onion is just beginning to soften. Add the garlic and sauté for 1 minute, stirring constantly, until fragrant.

Add the chicken stock, shredded chicken, brown rice, sea salt, and pepper. Bring the soup to a boil, reduce the heat to maintain a rolling simmer, cover, and simmer for 20 minutes, or until the carrots and celery are just softened.

Right before serving, add the dill and simmer, uncovered, for 1 minute. Serve.

YIELD: 4 TO 6 SERVINGS

soup's on

Chowder without dairy? I know, it sounds strange. But many years ago, when my mom's gut was healing and wouldn't tolerate dairy, this version of chowder satisfied her soul. With this soup, it is best to prepare all the vegetables before beginning to cook, or the process stutters rather than flows (to prevent the raw potatoes from browning, place in a bowl with cold water to cover, and strain right before adding to the pot).

Spuds 'n Corn Chowder for a Crowd

12 ounces (336 g) bacon, roughly chopped

1 cup (160 g) finely diced sweet onion

1 cup (120 g) finely diced celery, leaves left on

1 cup (105 g) cleaned and thinly sliced leeks

2 tablespoons (20 g) minced garlic

8 cups (1880 ml) homemade chicken stock (page 82)

5 cups (750 g) fresh corn, cut from the cob, divided (about 5 large ears)

5 cups (550 g) peeled and medium diced Yukon gold potatoes, divided

1 bay leaf

3 teaspoons (18 g) sea salt, divided

1 teaspoon freshly ground pepper

¼ teaspoon cayenne pepper

¼ cup (16 g) chopped fresh flat-leaf parsley

¼ cup 25 g) diagonally sliced scallion, for garnish

In a large-size soup pot over medium heat, add the bacon pieces and cook until crisp, approximately 15 minutes, stirring occasionally. Transfer the bacon pieces with a slotted spoon to drain on paper towels. Set aside. Pour the bacon fat into a glass measuring cup with a pour spout.

Add 2 tablespoons (30 ml) bacon fat back to the soup pot over medium heat. Add the onion, celery, and leeks. Sauté over medium heat, stirring occasionally, for 5 minutes, until the onions are translucent. Add the garlic and sauté, stirring constantly, for 1 minute, until fragrant.

Add 1 cup (235 ml) of the chicken stock and, using a wooden spoon or spatula, scrape the brown bits from the bottom of the pan. Add the remaining 7 cups (1645 ml) stock, 3 cups (450 g) of the corn, 3 cups (330 g) of the potatoes, the bay leaf, 2½ teaspoons (15 g) of the sea salt, and the ground pepper. Cover and bring to a boil over high heat. Lower the heat to medium and maintain a rolling simmer for 20 minutes, until the vegetables are tender.

Remove from the heat and allow the soup to cool for 5 minutes. Discard the bay leaf. Add 4 tablespoons (60 ml) bacon fat to the pot. Using an immersion blender, purée the mixture in the pot until creamy and smooth. If using a regular blender, blend in batches, and then return to the pot.

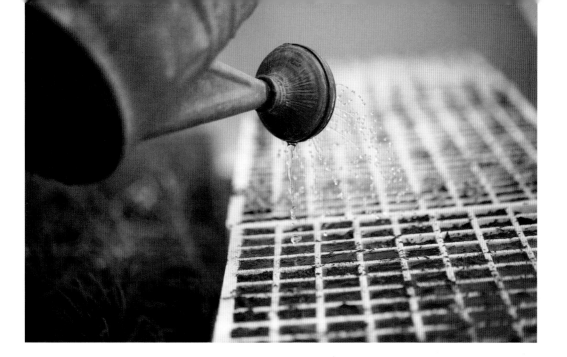

Add the remaining 2 cups (300 g) corn and remaining 2 cups (220 g) potatoes, along with the cayenne and parsley. Over high heat, return the soup to a boil. Lower the heat to medium and maintain a rolling simmer, uncovered, for 12 minutes, until the vegetables are cooked to al dente. Add the remaining ½ teaspoon sea salt. Stir to combine.

Serve warm, garnished with the sliced scallions and reserved crispy bacon.

YIELD: 6 TO 8 SERVINGS

RECIPE NOTE

Leeks grow in sandy soil, which gets trapped in the leek and requires careful washing. After slicing the leek, place the slices in a bowl of cold water. Stir gently to release the sand. Once the sand settles, lift out the floating slices and place in a colander to drain before using.

This recipe is a perfect one-pot meal. It is also quite simple to prepare—and did I mention gluten-free? In fact, the only grain in this soup is corn, whose omission would not compromise the recipe one bit.

Hearty Beef Soup with Brussels Sprouts

2 tablespoons (30 ml) bacon fat (page 33)

2 pounds (908 g) grass-fed stew beef, cut into bite-size chunks and thoroughly patted dried

½ cup (80 g) diced onion

½ cup (65 g) sliced celery, with leaves

1 tablespoon (10 g) minced garlic

8 cups (1880 ml) homemade beef stock (page 84)

2 cups (180 g) diced green cabbage

1 cup (130 g) sliced carrot

½ cup (65 g) frozen corn

2 cups (180 g) halved brussels sprouts

2 cups (260 g) fresh or frozen cauliflower florets (about 1 small head)

1 cup (120 g) diced zucchini (about 1 medium)

2 cups (360 g) diced tomatoes

½ cup (30 g) chopped fresh flat-leaf parsley

2 tablespoons (3 g) chopped fresh basil

In a large-size soup pot over medium-high heat, melt the bacon fat until it glistens. Add half of the meat in a single layer and let it cook undisturbed for 3 minutes, until browned. Use a spatula to flip the meat over. Repeat, browning the meat on all sides, then transfer to a plate and set aside. Add the remaining half of the meat and repeat the browning process. Once all the meat is browned, return it all to the pot and lower the heat to medium.

Add the onion and celery to pot and sauté for 5 minutes, stirring frequently, until softened. Add the garlic and sauté for 1 minute, stirring constantly, until fragrant.

Add 2 cups (470 ml) of the stock and use a spatula to scrape the browned bits from the bottom of the soup pot. Add the remaining 6 cups (1410 ml) stock and bring to a boil. Lower the heat to a rolling simmer. Cover and simmer for 1 to 4 hours; additional time simply yields more tender meat.

After simmering, add the cabbage and carrots to the pot. Bring to a boil. Cover, lower the heat to a rolling simmer, and simmer for 10 minutes.

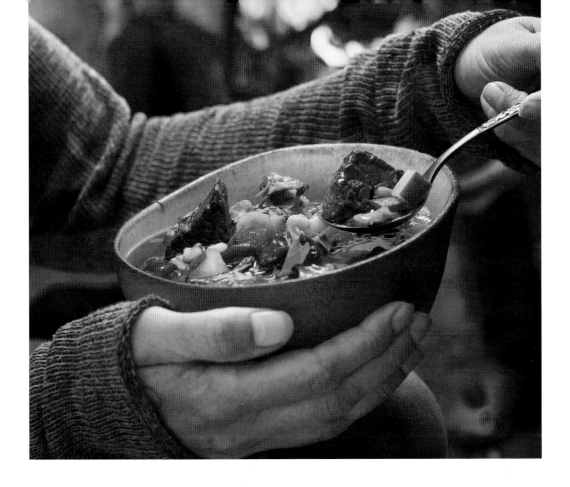

2 teaspoons (12 g) sea salt

1 teaspoon freshly ground pepper

2 dashes cayenne pepper, optional

5 ounces (140 g) roughly chopped
fresh spinach

After 10 minutes, add all the remaining ingredients except the spinach. Bring to a boil. Cover, lower the heat to a rolling simmer, and simmer for 20 minutes.

Right before serving, stir the fresh spinach into the simmering soup. Turn off the heat, wait 5 minutes, and serve.

YIELD: 8 TO 10 SERVINGS

This fresh recipe has a nice spike of heat that is rounded out with the last-minute addition of milk. If you would prefer a dairy-free recipe, go ahead and leave out the milk or replace with nut milk; however, the soup may be just a bit spicier. Don't forget to serve with the garnishes! The squeeze of lemon at the end makes the dish.

White Bean Chicken Chili

FOR CHILI:

2 tablespoons (28 g) butter

1 cup (160 g) finely diced yellow onion

½ cup (60 g) finely diced celery

1 cup (150 g) finely diced red bell pepper (about 1 small)

1 tablespoon (9 g) seeded and minced serrano pepper (about 1 medium)

3 cups (750 g) cooked Great Northern beans (page 52), divided

1 tablespoon (10 g) minced garlic

5 cups (1175 ml) homemade chicken stock (page 82)

½ cup (90 g) roasted, seeded, and medium diced poblano pepper (see Note at right)

2 cups (280 g) medium diced precooked chicken (page 32)

1 tablespoon (4 g) chopped fresh oregano

2 teaspoons (15 g) ground cumin

1 teaspoon chili powder

2 teaspoons (12 g) sea salt

½ teaspoon freshly cracked black pepper

½ cup (120 ml) milk

TO MAKE THE CHILI: In a large-size pot over medium heat, melt the butter until foaming. Add the onion, celery, red bell pepper, and serrano pepper. Sauté for 5 minutes, stirring occasionally, until the onion is just softened. While the vegetables cook, measure 1 cup (250 g) of the beans into a small-size bowl and mash with a fork.

Once the vegetables have sautéed for 5 minutes, add the garlic. Sauté for 1 minute, stirring constantly, until fragrant. Add the mashed beans, remaining 2 cups (500 g) whole beans, chicken stock, poblano, chicken, oregano, cumin, chili powder, sea salt, and black pepper. Stir to combine and bring to a boil. Cover, lower the heat to a simmer, and simmer for 20 minutes. Remove from the heat and stir in the milk. Season again, to taste.

TO SERVE: Serve each bowl topped with the diced avocado, fresh oregano leaves, and a drizzle of high-quality extra-virgin olive oil. Serve a lemon wedge next to each bowl to squeeze over the chili, just before eating.

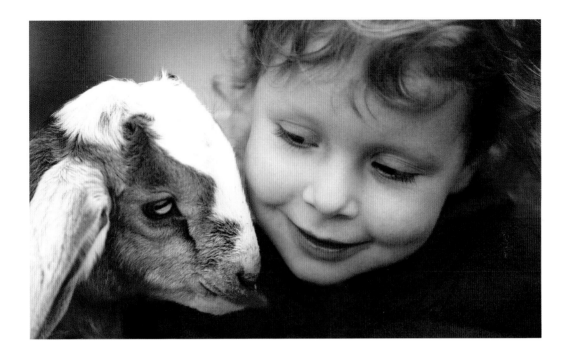

FOR GARNISH:

1 avocado, diced

Fresh oregano leaves

Extra-virgin olive oil, for drizzling

1 lemon, cut into 6 wedges

YIELD: 4 TO 6 SERVINGS

RECIPE NOTES

• To roast a poblano pepper, preheat the oven to 450ºF (230°C, or gas mark 8). Wash and dry the pepper thoroughly, then place on a cookie sheet. Roast for 20 minutes, turning the pepper with tongs every 5 minutes. The skin will be blackened and bubbled. Remove from the oven and use tongs to place in a glass bowl. Cover the bowl with plastic wrap or the lid of a pot, then leave for 5 minutes. Remove the pepper and place on a cutting board; peel off the skin. It should come off easily after being steamed in the bowl. Do not use water, which will wash away the flavor. Cut out the stem, slice lengthwise, and use a knife to scrap away the seeds. Dice the pepper and use!

• Our beans recipe (page 52) can be doubled for this dish.

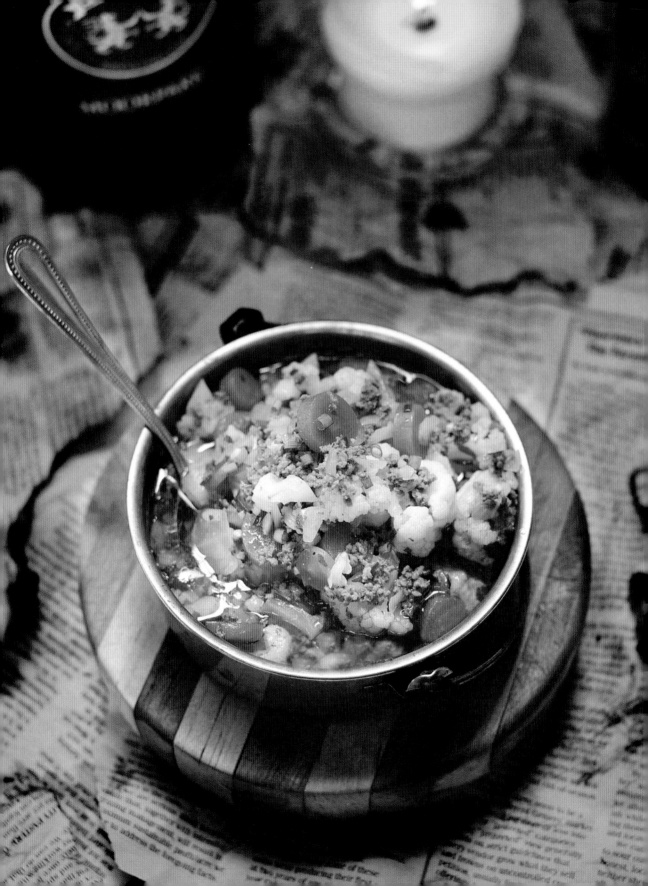

This comforting "stew" is actually a broth-based soup that has been a family mainstay for generations. Back in the day, "cheap" ground beef and a water base worked for my mom when too much month was left at the end of the money. Today, grass-fed beef and homemade stock elevate this dish in both nutrition and taste, while the cauliflower replaces the traditional potatoes, reducing the starch and increasing the flavor even more.

Poor Man's Stew

2 tablespoons (30 ml) ghee (page 22)

1 pound (454 g) ground beef

1 cup (160 g) diced red onion

1 tablespoon (10 g) minced garlic

6 cups (1410 ml) homemade beef stock (page 84)

¼ cup (12 g) chopped fresh chives

¼ cup (16 g) chopped fresh flat-leaf parsley

¼ teaspoon cayenne pepper

2½ teaspoons (15 g) sea salt, divided

½ teaspoon freshly cracked pepper, plus more to taste

2 cups (180 g) roughly chopped green cabbage

3 cups (390 g) peeled and thinly sliced carrot

3 cups (390 g) quarter-size cauliflower florets

YIELD: 6 TO 8 SERVINGS

In a large-size stockpot over medium-high heat, melt the ghee until it begins to foam. Add the meat and raise the heat to high. Using a potato masher, break up the meat. Continue to stir and break up the meat until it is fully browned, about 3 minutes. Lower the heat to medium and add onion. Cook for 3 minutes, stirring occasionally, until slightly softened. Add the minced garlic and sauté, stirring constantly, for 30 seconds, until fragrant.

Add 1 cup (235 ml) of the beef stock. Using a wooden spoon, scrape the sides and bottom of the pan to release the browned bits. Add the remaining 5 cups (1175 ml) broth, the chives, parsley, and cayenne, 2 teaspoons (12 g) of the sea salt, and the pepper. Raise the heat to high, cover, and return to a boil.

Add the cabbage and carrot, cover, and return to a boil. Lower the heat to medium and cook, covered, for 5 minutes.

Add the cauliflower, cover, and return to a boil. Lower the heat to medium-low and maintain a rolling simmer for 15 minutes, or until all the vegetables are fork tender. Add the remaining ½ teaspoon sea salt and additional cracked pepper, if desired.

I have made this chili for several chili cook-offs with much success. However, one year, I accidentally forgot to turn it down to a simmer and scorched the bottom! Too late for a new batch, I poured the chili into a new pot and served the burnt version with the name "Fire-Roasted Chili with Corn." And I came in third!

Cook-Off Chili with Roasted Corn

3 tablespoons (42 g) butter

1 cup (160 g) diced red onion

2 cups (140 g) sliced cremini mushrooms, optional

1 tablespoon (10 g) minced garlic

1 cup (150 g) diced red bell pepper (about 1 large)

¼ cup (36 g) seeded and diced jalapeño pepper (about 2 medium), optional

1 pound (454 g) ground beef

2 tablespoons (15 g) chili powder

1 tablespoon (7 g) ground cumin

⅛ teaspoon cayenne

2 teaspoons sea salt

½ teaspoon freshly cracked pepper

1 tablespoon (14 g) minced chicken liver, optional

1 can (28 ounces, or 784 g) fire-roasted crushed tomatoes

1 can (15 ounces, or 420 g) tomato sauce

3 cups (750 g) cooked kidney beans (page 52)

2 cups (260 g) roasted corn (see Note)

2 tablespoons (30 ml) cream

In a large-size pot, melt the butter over medium heat. Add the onion, mushrooms, garlic, red pepper, jalapeño pepper, and ground beef. Occasionally breaking up the meat with a wooden spoon, sauté for 10 minutes, until the beef is browned through and the mushrooms have softened and released their moisture.

Add the chili powder, cumin, cayenne, sea salt, pepper, and chicken liver, if using. Sauté for 1 minute so the dried spices can release their oils. Add the tomatoes, tomato sauce, and kidney beans. Cover and bring to a boil, then lower the heat to a simmer. Simmer, covered, for 1 hour, stirring occasionally. Remove the lid. Stir in the roasted corn and cream. Serve.

YIELD: 4 TO 6 SERVINGS

RECIPE NOTES

• Our beans recipe (page 52) may need to be doubled for this dish.

• To roast corn, preheat the oven to 400ºF (200ºC, or gas mark 6). While the oven is preheating, place 1 tablespoon (14 g) butter in a shallow baking pan and place in the oven for about 3 to 5 minutes to melt without browning. Place 2 cups (260 g) frozen or fresh corn cut off the cob on the tray. Sprinkle with ½ teaspoon salt and ¼ teaspoon pepper. Toss with a spatula to combine. Roast for 15 minutes, or until the corn is just beginning to brown.

• If fire-roasted crushed tomatoes are not available, use regular crushed tomatoes plus 2 teaspoons (10 ml) maple syrup.

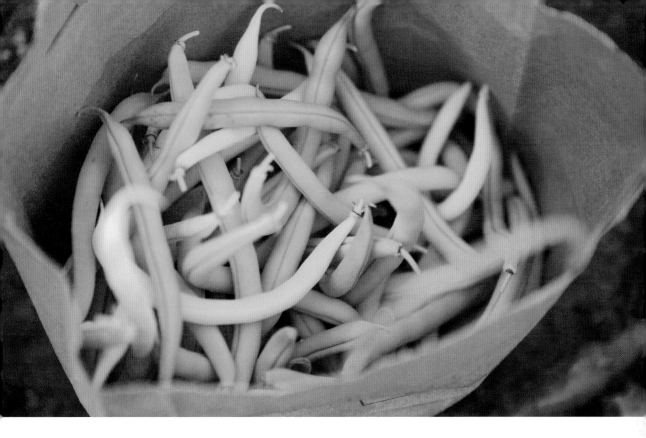

CHAPTER 8

A SALAD, PLEASE!

MY DEFINITION OF PERFECTION? Hearing the screen door slam shut as I take off toward the garden—basket hooked on my arm and my dog at my heels. After collecting a heaping pile of greens, beans, tomatoes, and herbs, I toss them with a bit of grass-fed cheese and a simple drizzle of oil and vinegar—that's perfection to me. That's abundance. It makes me feel rich, regardless of my bank account. Grow food and eat it—that's the good stuff of life.

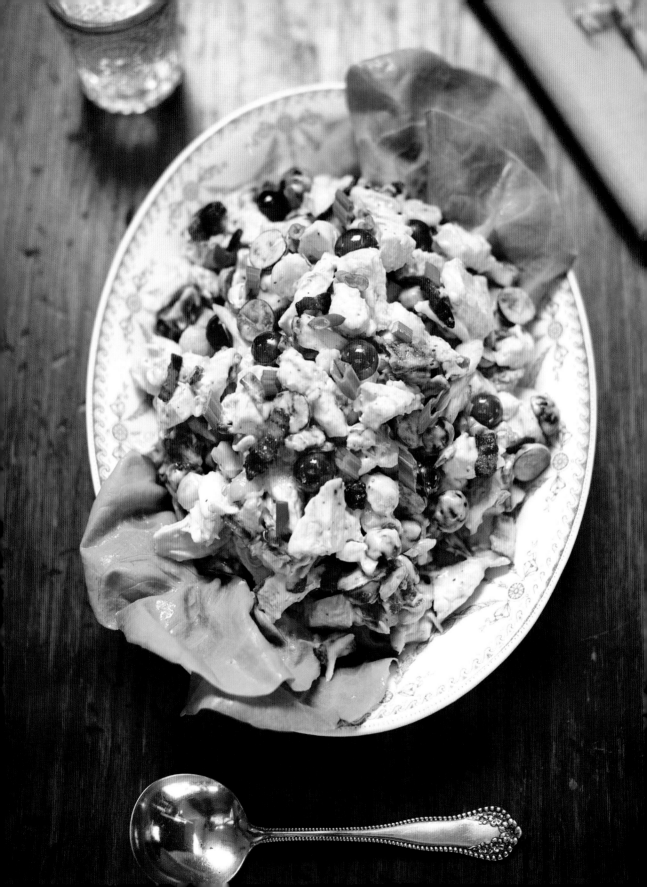

The first bold soul to combine fruit, chicken, and mayo should get a mighty high-five. Our homemade Simply Mayonnaise recipe (page 178) is an easy and valuable nutritional upgrade from store-bought, as it allows the cook to control the quality of oil used (and leave out the preservatives). Perfect for a gourmet sandwich or salad, crisp bacon and the deep flavor of dates take this classic dish over the top.

Classy Chicken Salad with Dates & Walnuts

3 cups (420 g) medium diced precooked chicken (page 32)

6 ounces (168 g) bacon, roughly chopped, cooked until crisp, and drained

½ cup (90 g) finely diced Medjool dates

¼ cup (25 g) thinly sliced scallion, both white and green parts

⅓ cup (30 g) finely sliced celery, cut on the diagonal

1 cup (150 g) seedless red grapes, halved

1 cup (225 g) Simply Mayonnaise Sweet Variation, chilled (page 178)

1 teaspoon sea salt

½ cup (68 g) crunchy macadamia nuts, roughly chopped (page 49)

YIELD: 4 TO 6 SERVINGS

Place the chicken, bacon, dates, scallion, celery, and grapes in a medium-size glass mixing bowl. Stir to combine. Pour the mayonnaise on top and sprinkle with the sea salt. Toss to combine, making sure to coat all ingredients well. Refrigerate until chilled, adding the nuts just prior to serving, but after the salad is chilled (to keep them crunchy).

RECIPE NOTES

• Freeze bacon for 30 minutes before chopping and cooking. This allows a sharp knife to slice through the meat easily.

• Chilling the salad causes some of the mayonnaise to be absorbed. You may have to "refresh" just prior to serving with a dollop or two more mayo. This is common and easy, and worth the effort.

We tire quickly of carrot and celery sticks, don't we? This raw salad is a wonderful and convenient solution. Before you begin, though, know that small, consistent dicing adds to the allure of this dish. And if you can find unfiltered and unpasteurized apple cider vinegar, buy it! Don't fear the pasteurization omission, which allows the "culture" (probiotics) to grow. Probiotics found in organic and raw foods help give the digestive system a much-needed boost.

Raw Chopped Salad

FOR DRESSING:

¼ cup (60 ml) apple cider vinegar

¼ cup (60 ml) unrefined flax oil

1 tablespoon (10 g) crushed garlic

⅓ cup (20 g) fresh chopped
   flat-leaf parsley

½ teaspoon poppy seeds

½ teaspoon sea salt

¼ teaspoon freshly cracked pepper

¼ teaspoon cayenne pepper,
   optional

FOR SALAD:

½ cup (80 g) finely diced sweet
   onion

½ cup (75 g) finely diced red bell
   pepper

½ cup (60 g) finely diced celery

½ cup (50 g) sliced green olives

½ cup (50 g) sliced sun-dried black
   or kalamata olives

1 cup (130 g) finely diced carrot

1 cup (120 g) finely diced zucchini

1 cup (120 g) finely diced yellow
   squash

1 cup (75 g) thinly sliced fresh snow
   peas

½ cup (50 g) small cauliflower florets

TO MAKE THE DRESSING: In a small-size glass jar with a tight-fitting lid, combine all the dressing ingredients. Shake well. Set aside, and allow the flavors of the dressing to marry while chopping the vegetables.

TO MAKE THE SALAD: In a large-size mixing bowl, combine all the salad ingredients. With a large-size spoon, stir well. Pour the dressing over the top and mix until thoroughly combined.

Chill in a covered glass container in the refrigerator until ready to serve.

YIELD: 6 TO 8 SERVINGS

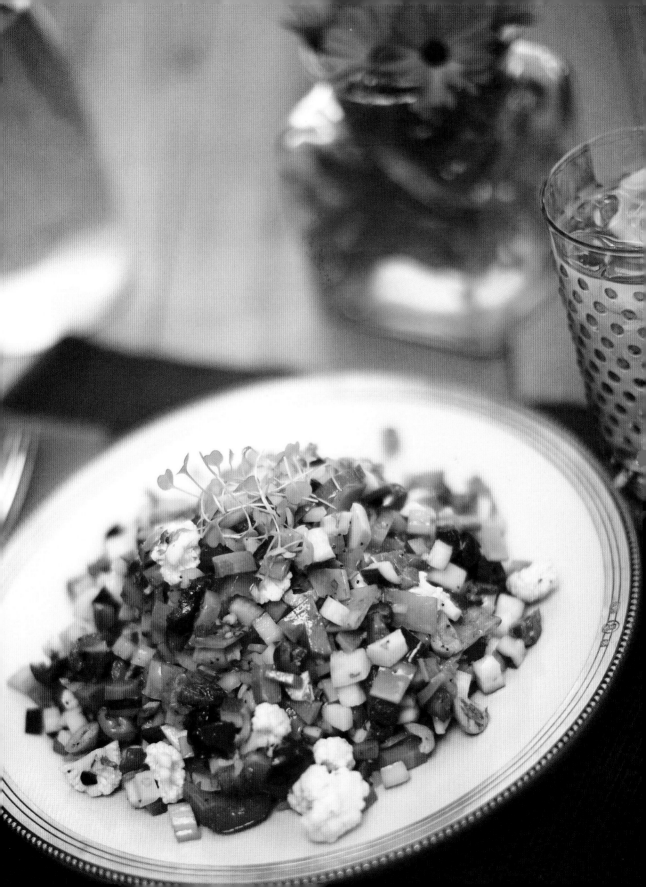

Caesar salad brings the controversy of raw egg into the equation. This recipe takes it back out! With the option of using raw egg or Dijon mustard, the cook can make the choice based on the company being fed and the ingredients available. When I have eggs from a farm I know and trust (such as Apricot Lane Farms!), I love the creaminess and decadence of the nutrient-dense raw egg version. And when I don't, Dijon mustard it is!

Caesar Salad with Sourdough Croutons

FOR CROUTONS:

3 tablespoons (42 g) butter

2 teaspoons herbes de Provence

¾ teaspoon sea salt

½ teaspoon freshly cracked pepper

3 cups (150 g) 1-inch (2.5 cm) wide cubed Rustic Sourdough Bread (page 186)

FOR DRESSING:

4 anchovies

2 tablespoons (30 ml) red wine vinegar

1 tablespoon (15 ml) lemon juice

1 teaspoon lemon zest

2 raw egg yolks, or 2 tablespoons (22 g) Dijon mustard

2 cloves garlic, peeled

½ cup (120 ml) extra-virgin olive oil

¼ cup (20 g) shredded Parmesan cheese

¼ teaspoon sea salt

½ teaspoon freshly cracked black pepper

TO MAKE THE CROUTONS: Preheat the oven to 350°F (180°C, or gas mark 4).

In a small-size pot over medium heat, combine the butter, herbes de Provence, sea salt, and pepper and heat until the butter is completely melted. Spread the sourdough cubes on a baking sheet in a single layer. Drizzle the melted butter mixture over the cubes and toss to coat, using your fingers to gently ensure each cube is covered with butter.

Bake for 10 minutes without turning or flipping. Remove the croutons from the oven and allow to cool. When completely cooled, store in a glass container with a lid until ready to use. If the croutons are not fully cooled when stored, they become soft. If this happens, re-toast briefly.

TO MAKE THE DRESSING: In a blender or food processor, combine the anchovies, vinegar, lemon juice, lemon zest, egg yolks, and garlic. Blend until the anchovies and garlic are incorporated. If necessary, scrape down the sides with a spatula. With the motor running, drizzle the olive oil through the opening. Turn off the blender and add the cheese, sea salt, and pepper. Pulse several times until incorporated.

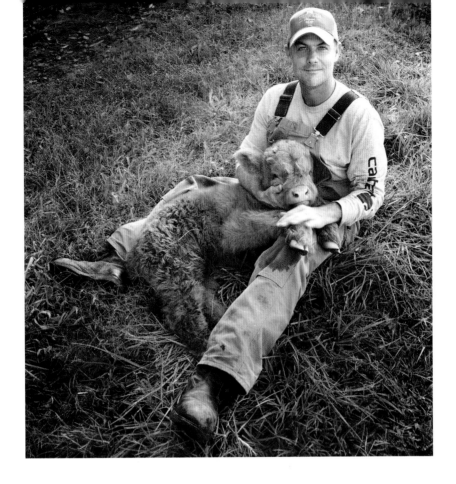

FOR SALAD:

6 cups (330 g) romaine lettuce cut into 1-inch (2.5 cm) pieces

½ cup (50 g) shaved Parmesan cheese

Freshly cracked pepper, to taste

YIELD: 4 SERVINGS

TO MAKE THE SALAD: In a large-size bowl, combine the romaine and croutons. Add 5 tablespoons (75 ml) dressing to the bowl. Toss and taste. Continue adding more dressing to suit your palate. The Dijon-based dressing will typically require more dressing than the egg-based version. Pour into a large-size serving bowl. Sprinkle the greens with the shaved cheese and freshly cracked pepper.

RECIPE NOTES

• To shave Parmesan cheese, use a vegetable peeler to peel the cheese into long, flat pieces, just like at a fancy restaurant.

• Be sure to zest your lemon before juicing—it is impossible the other way around! Also, choosing organic becomes very important when using the zest of a fruit, as a stronger concentration of pesticides is found on the skin.

a salad, please!

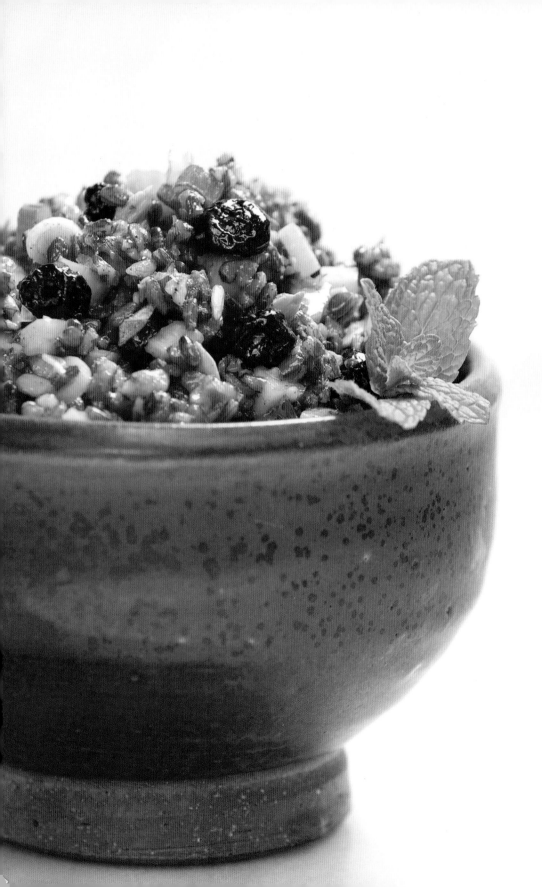

This sweet 'n tangy salad features a unique variety of heirloom rice—red rice—that is a deep and beautiful maroon hue. Heirloom, in layman's terms, is an antique seed that typically has more nutrition and unique qualities than many of today's mass-produced seeds. Several varieties of heirloom red rice are available in large grocery stores today, but when it's nowhere to be found, short-grain brown rice serves as a delicious substitute.

Red Rice Salad with Cumin Dressing

FOR SALAD:

3 cups (495 g) cooked red rice (page 54)

½ cup (55 g) coarsely chopped crunchy walnuts (page 49)

¼ cup (36 g) crunchy sunflower seeds (page 49)

½ cup (72 g) dried blueberries

¾ cup (90 g) finely diced celery

⅓ cup (35 g) thinly sliced scallion, both white and green parts

2 tablespoons (12 g) chopped fresh mint

FOR DRESSING:

¼ cup (60 ml) extra-virgin olive oil

2 tablespoons (30 ml) fresh lemon juice

2 tablespoons (40 g) raw honey (page 64)

1 teaspoon cinnamon

1 teaspoon cumin

¼ teaspoon nutmeg

1 teaspoon sea salt

¼ teaspoon freshly cracked black pepper

TO MAKE THE SALAD: In a medium-size bowl, combine all the salad ingredients. Toss gently and set aside.

TO MAKE THE DRESSING: In a small-size bowl or jar, combine all the dressing ingredients. Whisk well or shake.

Drizzle the dressing over the mixed salad and toss gently to incorporate. Chill for at least 1 hour before serving.

YIELD: 4 TO 6 SERVINGS

RECIPE NOTE

Look for dried blueberries that have been sweetened with apple juice concentrate rather than cane sugar. If dried blueberries can't be found, substitute currants, raisins, or dried cranberries.

This old family favorite appeals to all kinds of taste buds. It's a hearty dressing consisting of very basic ingredients—if you've got an onion in the pantry, chances are you can pull this off without a hitch. The dressing takes on a slight pink color when using a red onion. A sweet white onion, like a Vidalia, is a nice substitute and will result in a whiter dressing.

Sweet Onion Dressing >

½ cup (80 g) roughly chopped red onion (about 1 medium)
⅓ cup (80 ml) apple cider vinegar
¼ cup (40 g) honey granules (page 64)
1 teaspoon celery seed
1½ teaspoons powdered mustard
1 teaspoon sea salt
¾ cup (180 ml) extra-virgin olive oil

Place all the ingredients except the oil in a blender and blend until creamy.

Slowly drizzle the oil into the chute with the blender on medium speed. Continue to blend until the oil is incorporated.

Use immediately or refrigerate if not using the same day. Allow refrigerated dressing to warm to room temperature for 10 minutes before serving. Shake well before pouring.

YIELD: 1½ CUPS (355 ML)

Quick, classic, and delicious. Consuming raw honey from local beehives can actually help a body adjust to seasonal allergies. A cold dressing is a seamless way to add raw honey to the daily diet.

Balsamic Vinaigrette with Raw Honey

3 tablespoons (45 ml) balsamic vinegar
2 tablespoons (22 g) Dijon mustard
1 teaspoon minced garlic
1 teaspoon raw honey
¼ teaspoon sea salt
⅛ teaspoon freshly cracked pepper
½ cup (120 ml) extra-virgin olive oil

In a small-size bowl, combine all the ingredients except the oil.

Pour the oil into a liquid measuring cup, then slowly whisk into the balsamic mixture.

Use immediately or refrigerate if not using the same day. Allow refrigerated dressing to warm to room temperature for 10 minutes before serving. Shake well before pouring.

YIELD: ¾ CUP (180 ML)

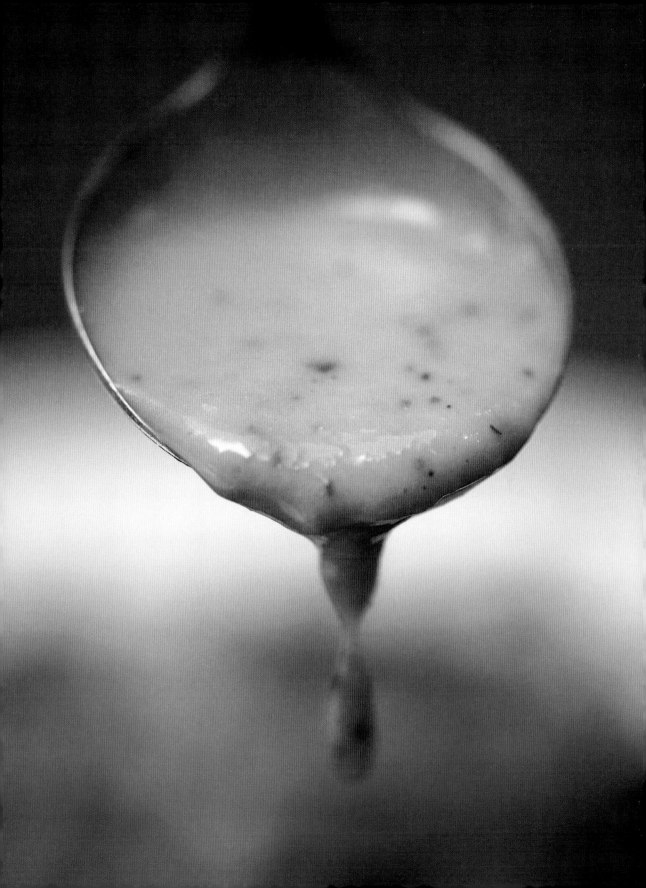

Look for a jam that is 100% fruit to avoid added sugar. Try different flavors for completely different results! Apricot is delicious for a salmon salad. Strawberry is lovely over a spinach salad with raw milk Cheddar.

Tangy Jam Dressing

3 tablespoons (60 g) all-fruit jam

2 tablespoons (30 ml) lemon juice

1 tablespoon (11 g) Dijon mustard

1 tablespoon (15 ml) apple cider vinegar

¼ teaspoon sea salt

⅛ teaspoon freshly cracked pepper

7 tablespoons (105 ml) extra-virgin olive oil

YIELD: ¾ CUP (180 ML)

In a small-size bowl, combine all the ingredients except the oil. Whisk to combine.

Whisk in the oil 1 tablespoon (15 ml) at a time, whisking until fully combined.

Use immediately or refrigerate if not using the same day. Allow refrigerated dressing to warm to room temperature for 10 minutes before serving. Shake well before pouring.

RECIPE NOTE

Try a creamy version, too. To make, simply stir a few tablespoons (45 g) plain yogurt into the original batch.

Living on a farm filled with fragrant lemon trees never gets old! This vinaigrette is a simple example why. In my case, I can easily collect the main ingredient on the 50-yard (45 m) "commute" from my office to the kitchen. Sure beats running to the grocery store!

Lemon Vinaigrette

¾ cup (180 ml) extra-virgin olive oil

½ cup (120 ml) fresh lemon juice (about 2 large)

¼ cup (60 ml) apple cider vinegar

3 pitted Medjool dates, roughly chopped

½ teaspoon sea salt

½ teaspoon freshly cracked pepper

Place all the ingredients in a blender. Blend until combined.

Use immediately or refrigerate if not using the same day. Allow refrigerated dressing to warm to room temperature for 10 minutes before serving. Shake well before pouring.

YIELD: 1½ CUPS (355 ML)

back to butter

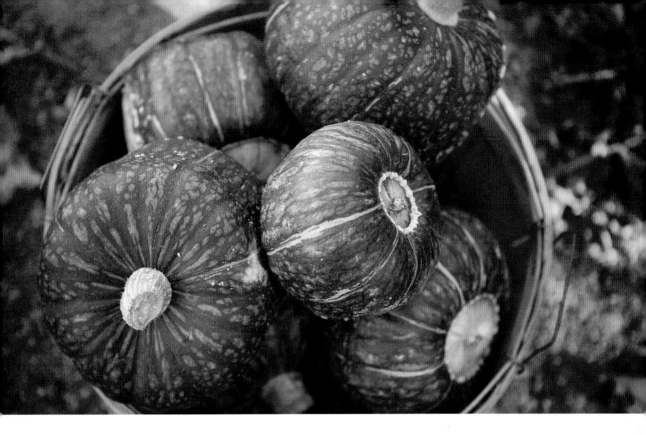

CHAPTER 9

NOURISHING SUPPERS

EVEN WHEN WE SEEM SO DIFFERENT—politics, race, religion, and so on—we all share the need to be fed. Through food, we bridge gaps. Simple nourishment gives us a source of conversation, a way to share, and a way to learn about each other's wants and needs. If you're ever in a conversation with someone and don't know what to say, ask them what kind of food they grew up eating for dinner, then just listen and learn. Food deserves a higher place in our hearts and on our priority lists. Let's spend more time talking about what we want for dinner. And when we can, *let's cook it at home.*

Scallops are delicious, "fancy," and take just minutes to cook. Growing up a vegetarian in landlocked Atlanta, Georgia, I spent my first few carnivorous years hesitant to dive into seafood. But after taking the scallop plunge, I was hooked. Here are a few tips for success: First, don't overcook them. Second, a hot pan is very, very important; they should release from the pan when they are somewhat firm and bouncy without being hard. And third, avoid crowding the pan. Cook in two batches, if necessary, dividing the oil between each. Try once or twice, and you will have this easy but upscale, entertaining-friendly dish mastered!

Seared Scallops with Creamy Carrot Purée

FOR PURÉE:

1 tablespoon (15 ml) extra-virgin olive oil

¼ cup (40 g) diced shallot

1 teaspoon minced garlic

2 cups (260 g) peeled and thinly sliced carrots

½ cup (120 ml) water

½ teaspoon sea salt, plus more to taste

A generous pinch of cayenne pepper

½ cup (120 ml) freshly squeezed orange juice

1 tablespoon (14 g) butter

TO MAKE THE PURÉE: In a large-size cast-iron skillet over medium-low heat, warm the oil until glistening, then add the shallots. Sweat the shallots for 3 minutes, stirring occasionally, until softened. Add the garlic and cook for 1 minute, until fragrant.

Add the carrots, water, sea salt and cayenne. Raise the heat to bring the liquid to a boil, then lower the heat to medium-low to maintain a rolling simmer. Cover and cook for 10 minutes, until the carrots are softened. Carefully pour the sauce into a blender. Add the orange juice and blend until creamy. Pour the sauce into a small-size saucepan (you'll use the cast-iron skillet for the scallops) over low heat and add the butter, stirring until melted. Re-season with sea salt to taste. Keep over low heat while cooking the scallops.

TO MAKE THE SCALLOPS: Wipe the cast-iron skillet with a paper towel. Evenly sprinkle the tops of the scallops with ¼ teaspoon of the sea salt and ¼ teaspoon of the pepper.

Over medium-high heat, heat ghee and garlic until the ghee is very hot but not smoking; the ghee will be glistening and the garlic will be sizzling fairly aggressively.

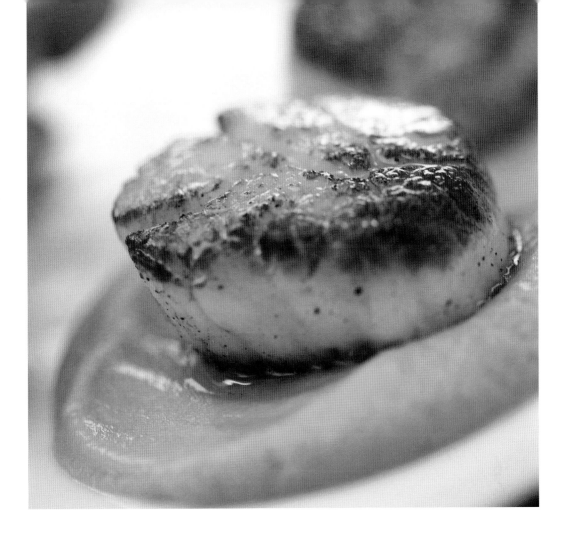

FOR SCALLOPS:

12 large sea scallops (about 1 pound
[454 g]), thoroughly patted dried
and brought to room temperature

½ teaspoon sea salt, divided

½ teaspoon freshly cracked pepper,
divided

3 tablespoons (45 ml) ghee
(page 22)

1 clove garlic, peeled and smashed

Add the scallops to the hot pan, seasoned side down, and
remove and discard the garlic clove, which has done its work by
flavoring the ghee. Sauté for 2 minutes, seasoning the tops with
the remaining ¼ teaspoon sea salt and ¼ teaspoon pepper.

After 2 minutes, flip the scallops with tongs; they should
release easily. Sauté an additional 2 minutes, until firm and
slightly opaque, but not hard.

Spread the carrot purée onto 4 plates and top with 3 scallops
each. Serve warm.

**YIELD: 4 SERVINGS, WITH 1½ CUPS
(355 ML) CARROT PURÉE**

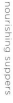

nourishing suppers

Store-bought salmon cakes are often made with bread crumbs, making them off-limits for those with a wheat or gluten allergy. Millet is a welcome grain alternative and works perfectly in these cakes. It can be found in health food stores and even some regular grocery stores. And if you wind up with any leftover cooked grain, it is delicious warmed with butter, cinnamon, berries, honey, and raw milk for breakfast.

Millet Salmon Cakes with Creamy Dipping Sauce

FOR DIPPING SAUCE:

1 cup (225 g) Homemade Crème
  Fraîche (page 45)

¼ cup (25 g) thinly sliced scallion,
  both white and green parts

¼ teaspoon lemon zest

2 tablespoons (30 ml) fresh
  lemon juice

¼ teaspoon Dijon mustard

½ teaspoon sea salt

¼ teaspoon black pepper

½ teaspoon cayenne pepper,
  or to taste

FOR SALMON CAKES:

7 tablespoons (98 g) butter, divided

½ cup (80 g) finely diced red onion

½ cup (80 g) finely diced fennel

½ cup (60 g) finely diced celery

¼ cup (15 g) chopped fresh flat-leaf
  parsley

1 pound (454 g) salmon, skinned
  and steamed or poached

TO MAKE THE SAUCE: Combine the sauce ingredients in a small-size bowl, mixing until well blended. Refrigerate until chilled and ready to serve.

TO MAKE THE SALMON CAKES: Preheat the oven to 350ºF (180ºC, or gas mark 4).

In a large-size cast-iron skillet over medium heat, melt 2 tablespoons (28 g) of the butter. Add the onion, fennel, and celery. Sauté for 5 minutes, stirring occasionally, until softened. Remove from the heat, stir in the parsley, and set aside to cool for 5 minutes.

Using clean hands, flake the salmon into a large-size bowl, being careful to remove any bones. Set aside.

In a separate bowl, toss the cooked millet with the ground flaxseed until the millet is coated. Add the millet mixture, walnuts, and cooled sautéed vegetables to the salmon, without mixing, and set aside.

In a small-size bowl, whisk together the sea salt, pepper, lemon zest, Dijon mustard, and eggs. Pour over the salmon mixture and gently toss together with a fork to combine. Using ⅓ cup (80 g) measurement, measure out and form 12 salmon cakes, wetting your hands to prevent sticking, if necessary. Set aside.

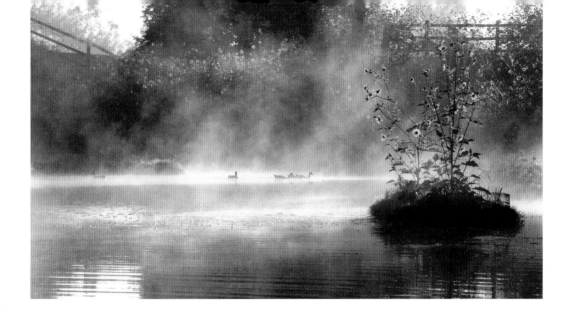

2 cups (370 g) cooked millet
    (page 53)
¼ cup (32 g) ground flaxseed
½ cup (55 g) chopped crunchy
    walnuts (page 49)
2 teaspoons sea salt
1 teaspoon black pepper
1 teaspoon lemon zest
1 tablespoon (11 g) Dijon mustard
3 eggs

**YIELD: 4 TO 6 SERVINGS, WITH 1 CUP
(225 G) SAUCE**

Line a regular sheet pan with parchment paper. Melt 2 tablespoons (28 g) of the butter and brush evenly onto the parchment paper. Set aside.

In the same large-size cast-iron skillet used for the vegetables (no need to clean it), melt 2 tablespoons (28 g) of the butter over medium heat. Add 6 salmon patties to the pan and sauté for 4 minutes, until the bottoms are lightly browned. Using a spatula and clean fingers (on the side of the cake that's still cool!), gently flip the cakes, browned side up, onto the buttered sheet pan and set aside. Repeat with the remaining 6 cakes and the remaining 1 tablespoon (14 g) butter. Add those, browned side up, to the sheet pan as well. Bake for 10 minutes.

Serve warm with the chilled sauce on the side.

RECIPE NOTE

I ask my fishmonger to skin and steam the salmon for me, which makes this a perfect weeknight meal. However, poaching fish at home is easy, too. First remove the skin, then fill a large-size pot halfway with water and 1 tablespoon (18 g) sea salt. Bring the water to barely a simmer; occasional bubbles will float to the surface, but the water will not be bubbly. Add the salmon, maintain a low simmer, and cook for 25 minutes. Remove the fish and drain well in a colander.

nourishing suppers

Sea bass is a deliciously moist fish that is difficult to overcook. It's also a decadent and somewhat expensive fish, making it a very special main dish. Sea bass was overfished for years, causing it to be pulled from many sustainably minded restaurants. Now it is strictly regulated, so always look for an MSC (Marine Stewardship Council) certification when purchasing your fish. The second key to this recipe is the homemade sourdough bread crumbs. Store-bought bread crumbs will not substitute because the flavor and texture are unsuitable.

Fresh Herb–Crusted Sea Bass with Sourdough Bread Crumbs

2 tablespoons (30 ml) lemon juice

6 tablespoons (84 g) butter, divided

1½ cups (75 g) Sourdough Bread Crumbs (page 188)

¼ teaspoon lemon zest

¼ cup (12 g) chopped fresh chives

¼ cup (15 g) chopped fresh flat-leaf parsley

⅛ teaspoon cayenne

1 tablespoon (10 g) minced garlic

¾ teaspoon sea salt, divided

¾ teaspoon freshly cracked pepper, divided

1 egg, lightly beaten

1½ pounds (680 g) sea bass, skinned, deboned and cut into 4 to 8 pieces

YIELD: 4 SERVINGS

Preheat the oven to 350ºF (180ºC, or gas mark 4). In a 9 x 13-inch (23 x 33 cm) glass baking dish, combine the lemon juice and 3 tablespoons (42 g) of the butter. As the oven preheats, place the dish in the oven to melt the butter, approximately 5 minutes. Remove from the oven and set aside for 5 minutes to cool.

In a medium-size saucepan, melt the remaining 3 tablespoons (42 g) butter and set aside.

In another medium-size bowl, combine the bread crumbs, lemon zest, chives, parsley, cayenne, garlic, ¼ teaspoon of the sea salt, and ¼ teaspoon of the cracked pepper. Toss well with a fork to combine, making sure to break up the lemon zest, which tends to stick together. Pour the egg over the mixture and toss with a fork to combine. Pour the melted butter over the mixture and toss again. This is your topping.

Dredge both sides of each piece of fish in the lemon/butter mixture in the pan and lay the fish prettiest side up in the dish. Sprinkle the remaining ½ teaspoon sea salt and ½ teaspoon pepper evenly on the tops of the fish. Generously pile the top-

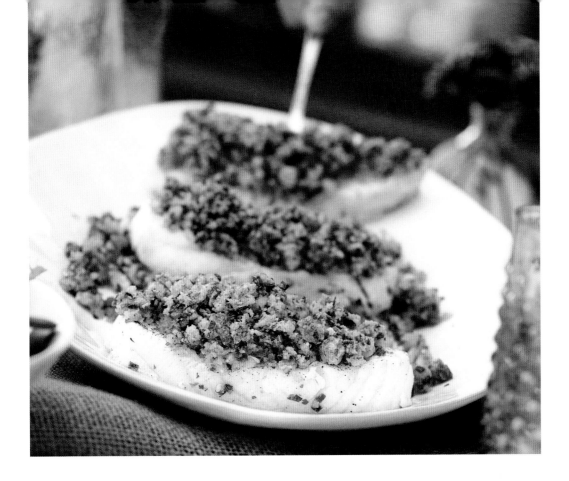

ping on each piece of fish, letting it fall to the sides. Sprinkle any extra in the pan alongside the fish.

Bake for 20 minutes. Test with a fork along the side of the fish. The fish should be moist and pull apart in large flakes. If not, return the fish to the oven, baking in 5-minute increments until ready. If the breading becomes too brown, tent the dish loosely with foil. Serve immediately.

RECIPE NOTE

If you didn't have your fish deboned by your fish monger, here's how to do it at home: Wash and pat the fish thoroughly dry with a paper towel. Run clean fingers down the fish to feel for the bones. Sea bass bones do not remove easily with tweezers like salmon bones do. Therefore, to remove the bones, cut neatly down both sides of the bones and remove the strip of bone entirely; some flesh may be sacrificed. If the bass started as one long piece, proceed to cut 4 even squares of fish. If your fishmonger cut the fish into 4 pieces (with bone) before purchase, removing the bones will result in 8 smaller pieces of fish. If this is the case, simply serve 2 pieces of fish per person.

This meal is a very versatile vegetable-based dish. Along with being served as a traditional rice and beans dish, the rice may be stirred into the finished beans and used as a filling for bean tacos. To serve, simply warm sprouted tortillas in the oven and provide fixings such as lettuce, avocado, mango, jicama, and sliced red peppers.

Coconut Black Beans & Brown Rice

1 tablespoon (14 g) coconut oil

1 cup (160 g) small diced red onion

1½ cups (225 g) small diced yellow pepper (about 1 large)

¼ cup (36 g) seeded and minced jalapeño (about 3 large)

1 tablespoon (10 g) minced garlic

1 tablespoon (6 g) minced fresh ginger

1 teaspoon ground coriander

⅛ teaspoon cayenne pepper, optional

5 cups (860 g) cooked black beans (page 52)

1 can (13½ ounces, or 378 ml) whole coconut milk

2½ teaspoons (15 g) sea salt

1 teaspoon raw honey

1 tablespoon (15 ml) freshly squeezed lime juice

3 cups (495 g) cooked long-grain brown rice (page 54), warmed

1 mango, peeled and sliced, for garnish

1 avocado, peeled, pitted, and sliced, for garnish

In a large-size saucepan with tall sides over medium heat, melt the coconut oil until glistening. Add the onion and yellow pepper and sauté for 5 minutes, stirring occasionally, until softened. Add the jalapeño, garlic, ginger, coriander, and cayenne. Sauté for 2 minutes, stirring constantly, until fragrant.

Add the beans and coconut milk, stirring to combine, and bring to a boil over high heat. Lower the heat to medium and boil gently for 10 minutes, stirring occasionally, while the sauce thickens. Remove from the heat and stir in the sea salt, honey, and lime juice. Serve warm over brown rice with mango and avocado for garnish.

YIELD: 4 TO 6 SERVINGS

RECIPE NOTE

To mince ginger, use the side of a spoon or a paring knife to peel or cut away the skin of the gingerroot. Then, using a sharp knife, very finely chop the ginger. A microplane zester also works very well for this purpose.

The bone broth in this dish turns a versatile sauce into one that is also very health supportive. Use with any recipe calling for marinara or try it in our Mushroom Marinara over Roasted Spaghetti Squash (page 122). It's also the perfect recipe to make using homemade jarred tomatoes from last summer's garden, if you have them! Otherwise, look for tomatoes packaged in glass. If you can only find canned, try to find a company that is careful about eliminating BPA (Bisphenol A), an endocrine-disrupting chemical, from the linings of their cans (page 217).

Bone Broth Marinara

2 tablespoons (28 g) butter

1½ cups (240 g) diced yellow onion

1 tablespoon (10 g) minced garlic

2 tablespoons (6 g) Italian seasoning

½ teaspoon fennel seeds, crushed

1½ teaspoons sea salt

1 teaspoon freshly cracked pepper

1 cup (235 ml) homemade chicken stock (page 82)

1 jar or can (28 ounces, or 784 g) fire-roasted crushed tomatoes

1 jar or can (28 ounces, or 784 g) tomato purée

1 teaspoon maple syrup

2 teaspoons (10 ml) apple cider vinegar

YIELD: 8 CUPS (1960 G)

In a large-size pot, melt the butter over medium heat. Add the onion and sauté for 5 minutes, stirring occasionally, until softened. Add the garlic and sauté for 1 minute, stirring occasionally, until fragrant.

Add the Italian seasoning, fennel, sea salt, and pepper. Sauté for 1 minute, while stirring constantly, to release the flavor of the dried spices. Add the chicken stock, crushed tomatoes, tomato purée, maple syrup, and apple cider vinegar. Stir to combine. Bring to a boil. Lower the heat to medium and simmer, uncovered, for 50 minutes. Adjust the heat to maintain a rolling simmer, stirring occasionally.

RECIPE NOTES

• To crush fennel seeds, use a mortar and pestle or roughly chop using a knife on a clean cutting board.

• Homemade Italian seasoning is easy to make! Simply combine 1 tablespoon (3 g) oregano, 1 tablespoon (2 g) marjoram, 2 teaspoons (2 g) thyme, 2 teaspoons (1.5 g) basil, 1 teaspoon (1.2 g) rosemary, and 1 teaspoon (1 g) sage.

The paleo diet, which has many crossovers to a traditional foods diet, has popularized using spaghetti squash in place of pasta for a range of comfort dishes, and for good reason. Variations on this dish are made at least twice a month in my house, and I'm always left feeling full without feeling heavy.

Mushroom Marinara over Roasted Spaghetti Squash

FOR SPAGHETTI SQUASH:

2½ pounds (1135 g) spaghetti squash

2 tablespoons (28 g) butter

½ teaspoon sea salt

½ teaspoon freshly cracked pepper

FOR MARINARA:

2 tablespoons (36 g) sea salt

2 cups (140 g) bite-size broccoli florets

2 tablespoons (28 g) butter

1 cup (160 g) diced red onion

1 tablespoon (10 g) minced garlic

1 pound (454 g) cremini mushrooms, thinly sliced

1 tablespoon (4 g) chopped fresh oregano

1½ teaspoons (9 g) sea salt

½ teaspoon pepper

3 cups (735 g) Bone Broth Marinara (page 121)

½ cup (50 g) pitted kalamata olives

½ cup (50 g) grated Parmesan cheese, optional, for garnish

TO MAKE THE SPAGHETTI SQUASH: Preheat the oven to 400ºF (200ºC, or gas mark 6). Wash the squash and cut lengthwise from root to stem. Scoop out the seeds, stopping before the flesh of the squash, which will be stringy.

In a roasting pan with a rack, place the squash cut-side down on the rack. Pour approximately 4 cups (940 ml) water into the bottom of the pan to reach a ½-inch (1.3 cm) depth.

Carefully place the pan into the hot oven and bake for 1 hour, or until a fork pierces through the skin and the flesh with slight resistance and an indentation remains when pressed, though the squash should not be mushy. Remove from the oven and, using a fork or tongs, place the spaghetti squash cut-side up on a cutting board. Into each cavity, place 1 tablespoon (14 g) butter and sprinkle each with ¼ teaspoon sea salt and ¼ teaspoon pepper. Allow the squash to cool for 5 minutes and melt the butter. Using a fork, shred the squash into a large-size serving bowl and set aside. The "noodles" will be al dente.

TO MAKE THE MARINARA: In a medium-size pot over high heat, bring 10 cups (2350 ml) water and the sea salt to a boil. Add the broccoli florets and blanch for 45 seconds. Using a slotted spoon, scoop the florets out of the boiling water and into a mesh strainer. Run under cold water for 30 seconds to stop the cooking process. Strain well and set aside.

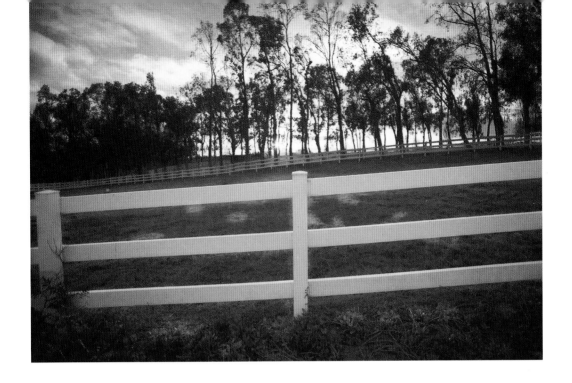

In a large-size sauté pan with tall sides over medium heat, melt the butter until foaming. Add the onion and sauté for 5 minutes, stirring occasionally, until softened. Add the garlic and mushrooms and sauté for 20 minutes, stirring occasionally, until the mushrooms have softened and the water released from the mushrooms has evaporated.

Add the oregano, sea salt, and pepper. Stir to combine, then add marinara and olives and stir again. Continue to cook until heated through.

Gently pour the marinara over the top of the spaghetti squash. Garnish with the broccoli florets and Parmesan cheese. Serve immediately.

YIELD: 4 SERVINGS

RECIPE NOTE

To prepare mushrooms, wipe with a damp cloth or paper towel. Trim the very bottom of the stem and slice vertically down through both the stem and the cap.

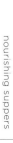

This meal (pictured on page 66) is an interactive, build-your-own dinner that has always been a staple in our house. It's so easy and fun! Simply make a batch of perfect baked potatoes, whip up the cheese sauce, and select as many toppings as you'd like from our lists below. Set everything out, and let your family create! My mom remembers hoping as a little girl to be given the extra skin from my Gramma's baked potato. I plainly see a miniature version of my mom with big ol' eyes of anticipation as she watched Gram scoop out the steaming pulp and slide a chunk of real butter into that perfect vegetable cup.

Baked Potatoes with the Works

FOR POTATOES:

4 large russet potatoes (or variety of
   choice)

4 teaspoons melted lard (page 23)
   or melted ghee (page 22)

Sea salt of choice: lemon pepper,
   garlic, or regular

Freshly cracked black pepper

1 recipe Foolproof Cheese Sauce
   (page 46)

MEAT OPTIONS:

Cook-Off Chili with Roasted
   Corn (page 100)

Bacon

Sausage

Pancetta

RAW VEGETABLE OPTIONS:

Fresh corn cut from the cob

Diced onion

Sliced scallion

Diced avocado

TO MAKE THE POTATOES: Several hours before dinner preparation, scrub the potatoes and set aside to thoroughly dry. If in a hurry, take care to thoroughly pat the potatoes dry after washing, or let the potatoes spend a minute or two in the preheating oven to hurry this process. You just want to start the preparation with a potato whose skin is clean and dry. Use a paring knife to cut any bad spots from the potatoes.

Preheat the oven to 400ºF (200ºC, or gas mark 6). Have ready an 8 x 8-inch (20 x 20 cm) or 7 x 11-inch (17.8 x 28 cm) glass baking dish. Use clean fingers to coat the skin of each potato with lard or ghee, liberally covering any exposed potato flesh. Set in the baking dish and liberally sprinkle with the sea salt and pepper.

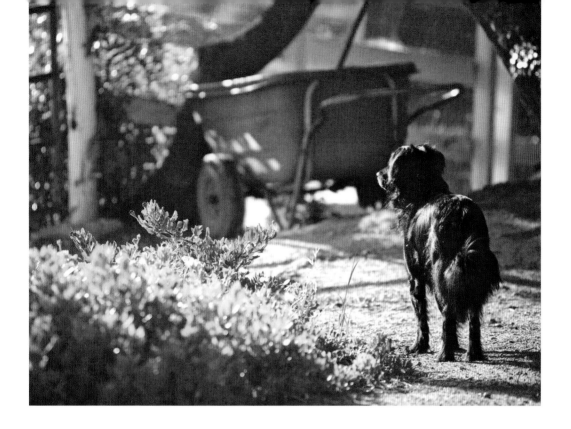

COOKED VEGETABLE OPTIONS:

Sautéed sliced mushrooms

Crispy sautéed onions

Steamed or roasted broccoli
or cauliflower

Sautéed chopped zucchini and
yellow squash

Roasted or sautéed sliced
fennel

GARNISH OPTIONS:

Salsa

Crème fraîche (page 45)

Butter

YIELD: 4 SERVINGS

Bake the potatoes for 1 hour. Test with a paring knife; it should slide into the center of the potato with ease after piercing the skin. If not fully baked, continue baking in 15-minute increments until done.

To serve, split the potatoes lengthwise, then top with a scoop of cheese sauce and the desired toppings.

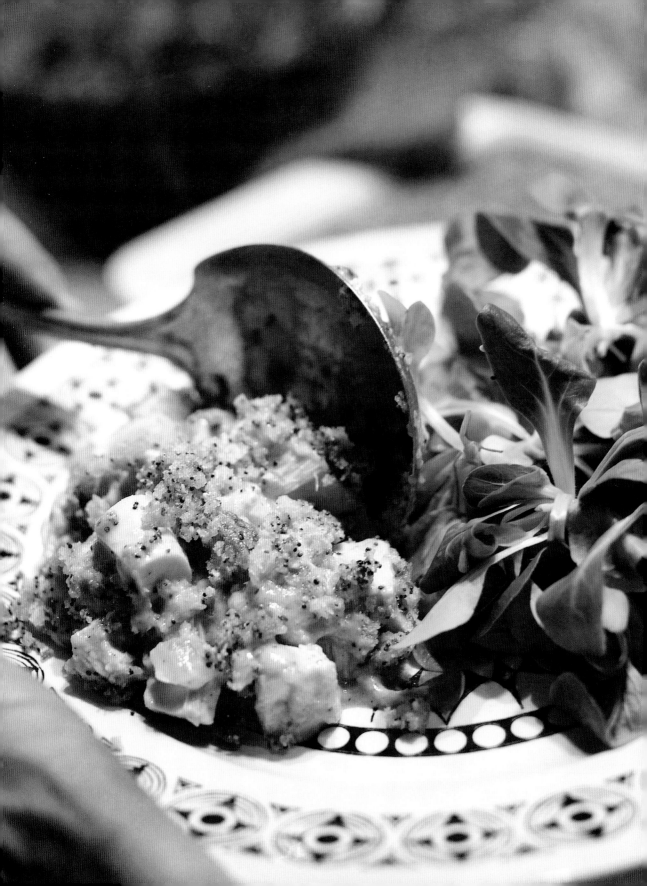

There's a good chance you remember this comfort food dish of the 1980s. My mom would make several batches at a time, in order to feed my hungry, basketball-playing brother and his teammates. Filled with processed foods at that time, we've since reinvented it with sprouted flour and a simple homemade gravy. Just like before, only better.

The New Poppy Seed Chicken Casserole

FOR CASSEROLE BASE:

5 cups (700 g) packed medium-diced precooked chicken (page 32)

4 tablespoons (56 g) butter

½ cup (80 g) finely diced yellow onion

6 tablespoons (45 g) fresh-milled, sprouted, whole wheat pastry flour (page 55)

2 cups (470 ml) homemade chicken stock (page 82)

1 teaspoon sea salt

½ teaspoon freshly cracked black pepper

¾ teaspoon poultry seasoning

½ cup (112 g) sour cream

FOR TOPPING:

3 tablespoons (42 g) butter

1½ cups (75 g) Sourdough Bread Crumbs (page 188)

½ cup (50 g) finely grated Parmesan

1 tablespoon (11 g) poppy seeds

YIELD: 4 TO 6 SERVINGS

TO MAKE THE CASSEROLE BASE: Preheat the oven to 350°F (180°C, or gas mark 4). Spread the chicken in an ungreased 8 x 8-inch (20 x 20 cm) glass baking dish.

In a large-size sauté pan over medium heat, melt the butter until foaming. Add the onion and cook for 5 minutes, stirring occasionally, until softened. Sprinkle the flour over the onion. Whisk for 2 minutes, then slowly add the chicken stock, whisking to incorporate. Whisk in the sea salt, pepper, and poultry seasoning. Bring to a boil over high heat, then lower the heat to medium-high and cook, whisking constantly, for 2 minutes, or until thickened. Remove from the heat and cool slightly.

TO MAKE THE TOPPING: In a small-size saucepan, melt the butter over medium heat. Set aside. In a medium-size bowl, combine the bread crumbs, Parmesan, and poppy seeds. Toss well to combine. Drizzle the butter over the top of the bread crumb mixture. Toss well to combine.

Now that the gravy has cooled slightly, whisk in the sour cream. Pour over the chicken in the baking dish and gently fold to coat. Crumble the bread crumb topping evenly over top.

Bake for 30 minutes. It's ready when the topping is light brown and the gravy is bubbling. Let stand for 5 minutes before serving.

Mom came up with this dish by accident. She turned down the heat on her baked chicken in order to play Cornhole with the neighbors and came home to find moist, fall-off-the-bone chicken!

Moist Oven Chicken

FOR CHICKEN:

2 bone-in chicken breast halves, skin on (1 breast, split)

2 bone-in chicken legs with thighs, skin on

3 tablespoons (45 ml) melted bacon fat (page 33), divided

2½ teaspoons (15 g) sea salt, divided

1½ teaspoons freshly cracked pepper, divided

4 cloves garlic, peeled

8 carrots (about 1 pound [454 g])

12 fingerling potatoes (1½ to 2 pounds [680 to 908 g])

FOR GRAVY:

¼ cup (60 ml) water

4 teaspoons arrowroot powder

1 cup (470 ml) homemade chicken stock (page 82)

Sea salt and pepper

YIELD: 4 SERVINGS

TO MAKE THE CHICKEN: About 2½ hours before dinner, preheat the oven to 325ºF (170ºC, or gas mark 3). Wash and thoroughly dry the chicken. Using a pastry brush and 1 tablespoon (15 ml) of the melted bacon fat, lightly oil the skin side of each piece of chicken. Evenly sprinkle this side with 1 teaspoon sea salt and ½ teaspoon pepper.

In a large-size oven-safe pan with an oven-safe lid (such as a Dutch oven), heat the remaining 2 tablespoons (30 ml) bacon fat over medium-high heat until it glistens. Carefully lay the meat, skin-side down, into the pan. While the meat is browning, using the melted oil in the pan, oil the other side of the meat with the pastry brush and sprinkle evenly with 1 teaspoon sea salt and ½ teaspoon pepper. Cook for 8 minutes, until nicely browned, then use tongs to flip the chicken. Sauté the second side for an additional 6 minutes. Remove from the heat, add the whole garlic cloves to the pan, cover, and place in the preheated oven. Bake the chicken, covered, for 1 hour.

While the chicken is baking, scrub the carrots and cut large carrots in half crosswise. Prep the potatoes by scrubbing, removing any "eyes" or bad spots. Soak the carrots and potatoes in a large-size bowl of cold water while the chicken cooks.

When the chicken has baked for 1 hour, drain the vegetables and add to the pan with the chicken. Season the vegetables with the remaining ½ teaspoon sea salt and ½ teaspoon pepper. Cook for 1 hour longer.

After 1 hour, test the vegetables for fork tenderness. If they are tender, remove the pot from the oven. If they are not, return

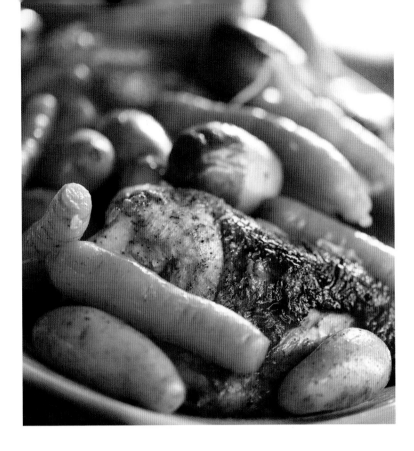

the pot to the oven and cook in additional 15-minute increments until the vegetables are fork tender.

Place the cooked chicken and vegetables on a large-size,
warmed serving bowl and re-cover with the lid from the
sauté pan.

TO MAKE THE GRAVY: Scrape the bottom of the now-empty
chicken pan and strain the juices into a small-size pot over
high heat, pouring off any clear fat.

In a small-size glass jar with a lid, combine the water and
arrowroot. Shake well and set aside.

Add the chicken stock to the pan juices. Bring the mixture to a
boil. Once boiling, lower the heat to medium and slowly add
the arrowroot mixture while constantly whisking. Simmer for
2 minutes, or until thickened. Season with sea salt and pepper
to taste.

Serve the chicken warm with the gravy on the side.

RECIPE NOTE

Arrowroot is an edible starch from the
root of a plant. Similar to cornstarch, it
can be added to water and stirred into
liquids to create thickening. Whereas
cornstarch is a common allergen,
however, arrowroot has been known
to actually calm the digestive tract.

nourishing suppers

This dish was first named Maple Dijon Chicken, but you'll see why it quickly became Sticky Chicken! Perfect for a cookout, football game, or casual dinner, it is delicious whether hot right from the oven or sliced cold and stuffed in a sourdough sandwich the next day. The sauce is rich and flavorful, and the meat is fall-off-the-bone moist. Kids love this meal.

Sticky Chicken

½ cup (112 g) butter

½ cup (120 ml) maple syrup

½ cup (88 g) Dijon mustard

4 teaspoons curry powder

2½ teaspoons (15 g) sea salt, divided

¼ teaspoon cayenne

4 bone-in chicken breast halves, skin on (2 whole breasts, split)

½ teaspoon freshly cracked pepper

YIELD: 4 SERVINGS

Preheat the oven to 350°F (180°C, or gas mark 4). Combine the butter, maple syrup, mustard, curry powder, 2 teaspoons (12 g) of the sea salt, and the cayenne in a 9 x 13-inch (23 x 33 cm) glass baking dish. While the oven is preheating, place the dish in the oven for 5 to 7 minutes, or until the butter fully melts but does not brown.

Remove the pan from the oven and whisk the ingredients to combine. Allow to cool for 5 minutes, then liberally dredge each piece of the chicken in the sauce. Gently slide your fingers between the skin and the flesh of the chicken, being careful not to tear the skin. Using a pastry brush, coat both the flesh and the skin thoroughly with sauce. Gently pull the skin back into place.

Arrange the chicken in a single layer in the pan, skin-side up. Sprinkle with the remaining ½ teaspoon sea salt and the pepper.

Bake, uncovered, for 30 minutes. Remove and baste with the pastry brush using the pan sauces. Bake, uncovered, for an additional 30 minutes.

Remove from the oven and preheat the broiler. Baste the chicken one final time, then broil for 2 to 3 minutes, until the chicken skin browns nicely. Be careful not to burn.

Cool for 10 minutes, then place on a serving platter. Whisk the pan juices and pour over the chicken. Serve!

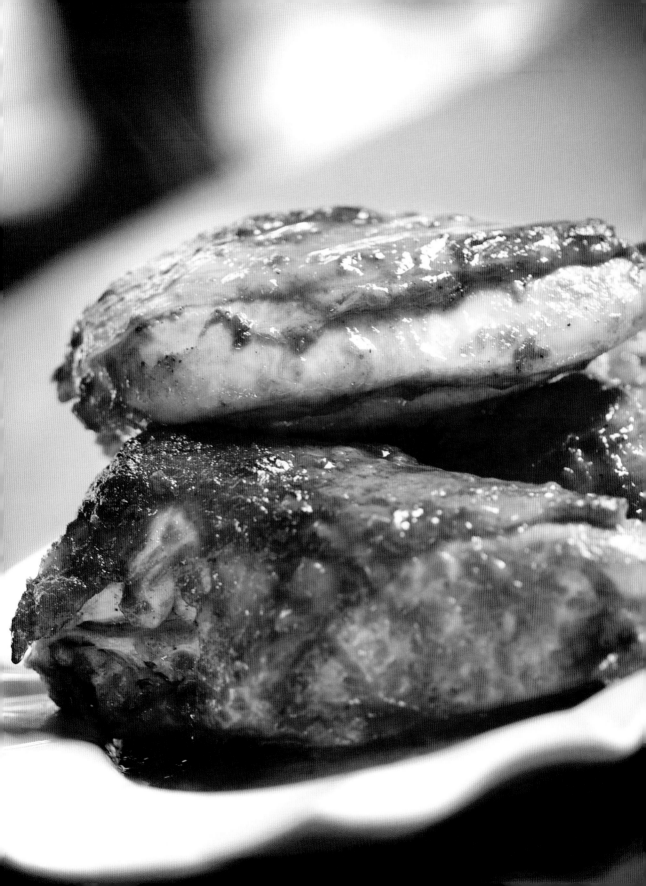

For more than forty years, our family has eaten a moist and unbelievably flavorful, oven-roasted turkey without the usual last-minute chaos. How? We roast our birds one or even two nights before—it makes Thanksgiving a breeze! Now, if your family prefers a bird cooked with stuffing, simply omit the celery, onion, and garlic, and substitute a favorite stuffing recipe. Note that you will need a large-size roasting pan, aluminum foil, parchment paper, a sterilized needle, and thread for this recipe.

Easy Holiday Turkey

20-pound (4.5 kg) turkey, defrosted
    if frozen
3 teaspoons (18 g) sea salt, divided
2 teaspoons freshly ground pepper,
    divided
3 celery stalks, cut into 4-inch
    (10 cm) pieces
1 full head unpeeled garlic, ¼ inch
    (6 mm) of top and bottom cut off
1 large yellow onion, peeled and
    halved
½ cup (120 ml) bacon fat (page 33)
2 quarts (2 L) homemade chicken
    stock (page 82)
2 quarts (2 L) homemade beef stock
    (page 84)

**YIELD: 14 TO 16 SERVINGS WITH PLENTY
OF LEFTOVERS**

Thanksgiving Eve (around 7 p.m.) or Thanksgiving Eve-Eve, preheat the oven to 400ºF (200ºC, or gas mark 6). Place a rack toward the bottom of the oven and remove the other racks (to fit the bird easily). In the bottom of the roasting pan, lay 2 long strips of heavy-duty aluminum foil along the center of each side, crossed like a plus sign. The strips will need to be long enough to cover the bird (like ribbons on a present). Rest a rack inside the roaster on top of the foil.

Wash and dry the bird. Season the cavity with 1½ teaspoons (9 g) of the sea salt and 1 teaspoon of the pepper. Place the celery, garlic, and onion into the seasoned cavity, and sew up both ends of the turkey with needle and thread.

Liberally coat the exterior of the turkey with the bacon fat and season with the remaining 1½ teaspoons (9 g) sea salt and 1 teaspoon pepper. Set the turkey, breast side down, on the rack. Cut a piece of parchment paper large enough to cover the top and sides of the turkey. Cover with parchment and close the foil strips up over the turkey and parchment, creating a tent. The turkey must be completely sealed in with no openings for heat to escape.

Roast for 1 hour, then lower the temperature to 250ºF (120ºC, or gas mark ½). Roast overnight or for a minimum of 12 hours. DO NOT PEEK! After 12 hours, carefully unwrap the foil and parchment, and lightly pull on one of the drumsticks, which, when ready, will easily pull away from the bird with a gentle twist. Until this is possible, continue roasting and checking in 1-hour increments, but be diligent about resealing the foil. Don't rush completion! Keep in mind that dinner is still many hours off!

When the turkey is fall-apart tender, remove from the oven, open the parchment-foil tent, and allow the meat to cool to the touch.

Preheat the oven to 350ºF (180ºC, or gas mark 4) (or just increase if it's still on). Remove the skin from the bird and set aside. Cut the turkey into pieces, being careful to keep the breast and drumsticks intact, and stack the meat into a cast-iron Dutch oven. Place the white meat on one side of the pot and the dark meat on the other for ease of serving. Use enough stock to completely cover the meat with equal parts chicken and beef stock. Place the lid on the pot and store in the fridge until 2 hours before serving.

Once the bird is in the fridge, arrange the skin in a single layer on a sheet tray. Roast in the oven for 30 minutes, turning the skin over after 15 minutes, until crispy. Let cool and store in a sealed container at room temperature.

Two hours before mealtime, warm the turkey. If the oven is occupied, simmer the covered pot over low heat until heated through. If the stove is occupied, place in a 300ºF (150ºC, or gas mark 2) oven until hot. Either option will make your home smell of roasted turkey, when in fact the turkey mess will have been cleaned up long ago!

When ready to serve, carefully lift the tender meat from the hot stock and place on a serving plate. Reserve the stock that's left behind for a great leftover turkey soup! Arrange the skin "cracklings" on the side of the plate. Serve and enjoy—without a messy kitchen!

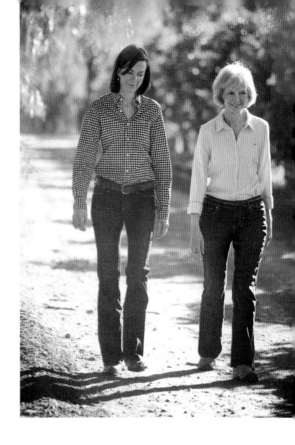

RECIPE NOTES

• As with all meats in this book, we strongly suggest local and pastured. It will make all the difference!

• Parchment paper is placed between the turkey and the aluminum foil here to limit aluminum exposure to the food. Aluminum cookware is a controversial topic that may or may not present a health risk, so we err on the side of caution.

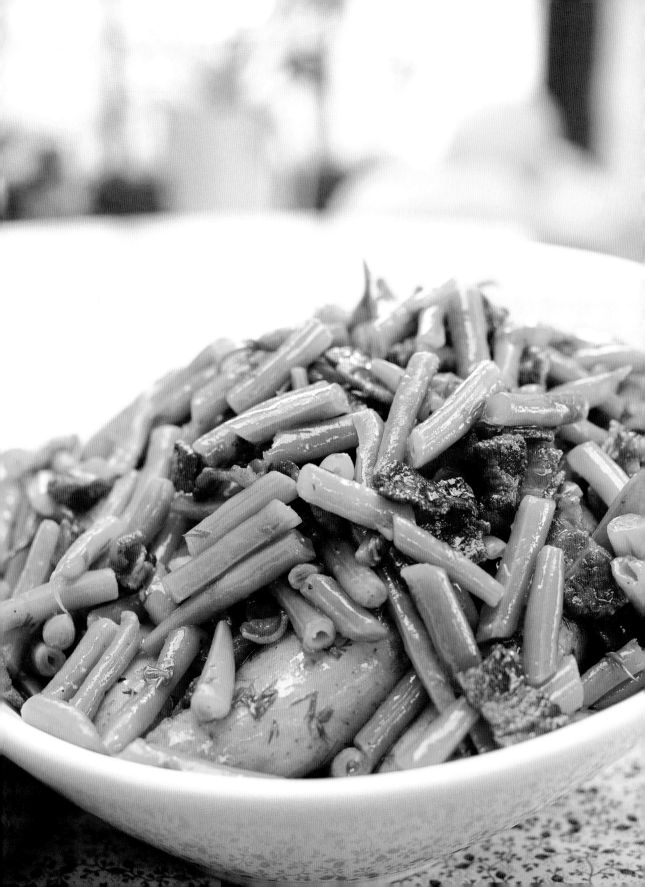

My aunt came up with this dish long ago based on summer's bounty. The fresh, spring taste of green beans and new potatoes are combined with the rich addition of bacon and butter to create a satisfying and comforting family dish. Start at the farmers' market and end with a happy family!

Aunt Mimi's New Potatoes, Green Beans, and Bacon with Dill

1 pound (454 g) bacon, cut into ½-inch (1.3 cm) pieces

3 tablespoons (54 g) sea salt, divided, plus more to taste

1½ pounds (680 g) fingerling potatoes, scrubbed, bad spots removed

7 cups (about 2 pounds [908 g]) fresh green beans, trimmed and cut into 1-inch (2.5 cm) pieces

3 tablespoons (42 g) butter

3 tablespoons (45 ml) extra-virgin olive oil

3 tablespoons (12 g) chopped fresh dill

2 tablespoons (8 g) chopped fresh flat-leaf parsley

Freshly ground pepper, to taste

YIELD: 4 SERVINGS

Fill a large-size pot with 3 quarts (2.7 L) water, cover, and bring to a boil.

While the water is heating, in a large-size sauté pan over medium-high heat, sauté the bacon until very crisp but not burnt, approximately 15 minutes. With a slotted spoon, remove the cooked bacon to drain on a paper towel. Reserve 3 tablespoons (45 ml) of the bacon fat.

Once the water has reached a boil, add 2 tablespoons (36 g) of the sea salt and the potatoes. Lower the heat to medium, cover with a lid, and boil for 5 minutes, then add the beans and remaining 1 tablespoon (18 g) sea salt. Raise the heat to bring back to a boil, then lower the heat to medium and boil for 15 minutes, or until the beans are crisp tender and the potatoes are fork tender (do not allow them to get past this).

While the vegetables are boiling, melt the butter in a small-size saucepan, then add the reserved bacon fat, olive oil, dill, and parsley. Stir to combine.

As soon as the vegetables are cooked, remove from the heat and drain in a large-size colander. Return the vegetables to the hot pot, then pour the butter mixture over the hot vegetables and carefully fold to distribute. Season to taste with additional sea salt and pepper. Sprinkle with bacon and serve.

I'd say this is the best pork tenderloin I've ever had. The marinade is delicious, but it's the layer of sweet onion that roasts beneath the tenderloin that sets the dish apart. Keep this dish in mind for entertaining!

Roasted Pork Tenderloin with Onion Marinade

FOR MARINADE:

1 tablespoon (10 g) minced garlic

¼ cup (40 g) grated sweet onion

1 teaspoon powdered mustard

¼ cup (60 ml) melted bacon fat (page 33)

2 tablespoons (30 ml) apple cider vinegar

1 pound (454 g) pork tenderloin

FOR TOPPING:

3 tablespoons (45 ml) ghee (page 22), divided

5 (¼-inch, or 6 mm) slices from the center of a sweet onion

¼ cup (40 g) diced sweet onion (use ends of above onion)

4 strips uncooked bacon, roughly chopped

1 teaspoon sea salt

½ teaspoon freshly cracked black pepper, plus more to taste

YIELD: 4 SERVINGS

TO MAKE THE MARINADE: In a zip-top bag, combine the marinade ingredients. Squeeze lightly to mix, and then add the tenderloin. Squeeze lightly to cover the meat. Seal the bag. Allow the meat to rest at room temperature for 1 hour. If you have more time, allow the meat to marinate in the refrigerator for up to 12 hours. Take the meat out of the fridge 1 hour before roasting to bring to room temperature, which allows the roast to cook evenly.

TO MAKE THE TOPPING: Preheat the oven to 425ºF (220ºC, or gas mark 7). In a 7 x 11-inch (17.8 x 28 cm) glass baking dish, add 2 tablespoons (30 ml) of the ghee. Place the dish in the oven as it preheats for 2 to 3 minutes, until the ghee is fully melted.

Remove the pan from the oven and line the onion slices down the middle of the pan in a single layer. Each slice should slightly overlap the next, creating a "roasting bed" for the tenderloin. Using a pastry brush, brush the tops of the onions with the melted ghee in the pan. Set aside.

In a small-size bowl, use a fork to toss the diced onion, bacon, sea salt, and black pepper. Evenly spread one-third of the bacon mixture across the top of the onion slices and set the rest aside.

Remove the tenderloin from the bag, leaving the excess marinade behind, and set on a plate.

In a large-size cast-iron skillet over high heat, melt the remaining 1 tablespoon (15 ml) ghee. Carefully add the tenderloin

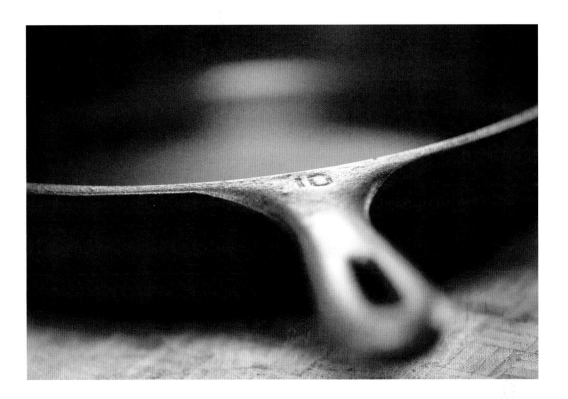

and quickly (1 to 1½ minutes per side) sear the meat on all sides until browned. Remove immediately and lay the tenderloin across the bed of onions. Carefully press the remaining bacon mixture on top of the seared tenderloin, allowing the excess to fall into the pan. Season one last time with a liberal amount of freshly cracked pepper, to taste.

Bake for 25 to 30 minutes, or until a meat thermometer inserted into the thickest part reaches 150°F (66°C). Pork is well done at 160°F (71°C), and will continue to cook during the next and final step, so take it out at 150°F (66°C) to avoid overcooking.

Remove from the oven, cover loosely with foil, and allow to rest for at least 5 minutes. Slice and serve with the extra bacon and onion topping heaped over the sliced tenderloin.

My great-grandma Scowden used to make this recipe years ago and it remains one of my mom's favorites. Like most everything, the dish has evolved—no more refined sugars, fresh pineapple replaces canned, and the sourdough bread crumbs are homemade. If you're feeling ambitious, try making homemade ketchup and mustard (pages 174 and 177) first!

Sweet Ham Loaf

FOR GLAZE:

½ cup (100 g) Sucanat (page 64)

1 tablespoon (15 ml) apple cider vinegar

1 teaspoon prepared yellow mustard (page 177)

1 tablespoon (15 ml) water

½ tablespoon (7 g) butter

FOR LOAF:

1 pound (454 g) ham, ground (see Note)

1 pound (454 g) ground pork

2 eggs, beaten

1 cup (50 g) Sourdough Bread Crumbs (page 188)

⅔ cup (160 ml) milk

2 tablespoons (30 g) ketchup (page 174)

1 cup (155 g) diced fresh pineapple

YIELD: 6 TO 8 SERVINGS

Preheat the oven to 325ºF (170ºC, or gas mark 3). Have ready a 2-quart (2 L) glass or ceramic ungreased loaf pan.

TO MAKE THE GLAZE: In a small-size pot, combine the Sucanat, apple cider vinegar, yellow mustard, and water over medium heat. Whisk well and simmer for 5 minutes. Remove from the heat, add the butter, and let melt. Stir to combine and set aside.

TO MAKE THE LOAF: In a medium-size bowl, combine the ham, pork, eggs, bread crumbs, milk, and ketchup. Using clean hands, gently mix to combine. Gently press the mixture into the loaf pan and top with the pineapple, lightly pressing the fruit into the loaf.

Cover with foil and bake for 30 minutes. Remove from the oven and increase the oven temperature to 350ºF (180ºC, or gas mark 4). Pour the prepared glaze over the loaf. Return the pan to the oven and bake for 1 hour, uncovered. When done, the loaf will pull away slightly from the sides of the pan and the topping will be browned and caramelized.

Remove from the oven and let rest for 10 minutes. Using two metal spatulas, lift the entire loaf from the pan. Slice and serve warm.

RECIPE NOTE

This is a perfect recipe to use up leftover ham from the holidays. Cut the ham into large chunks and place in the bowl of a food processor. Pulse approximately 25 times, until the meat has reached a uniform crumble.

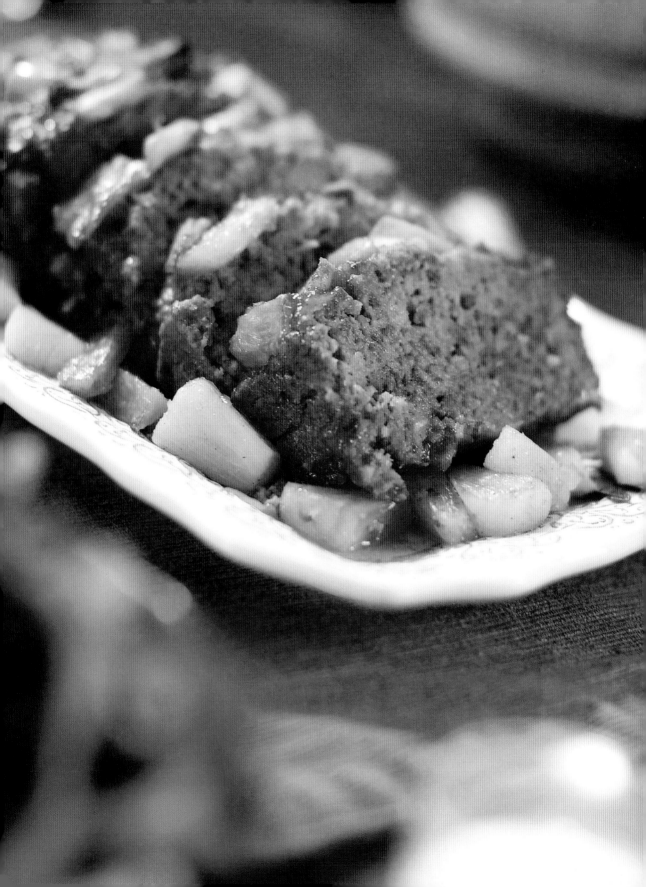

In this recipe, you will add one whole onion to the pot while it is simmering, only to subsequently remove and discard it, a unique technique that adds unbelievable depth of flavor to this one-pot dish. And though the total cook time of the dish is several hours, the active time is minimal and the result is comfort food at its finest!

Wonderful Winter Pot Roast Stew

2½ pounds (1135 g) rump roast

3 teaspoons sea salt, divided

1½ teaspoons freshly cracked
pepper, divided

1 tablespoon (15 ml) ghee (page 22)

2 tablespoons (28 g) butter

3 cups (480 g) medium diced onion

5 cups (1175 ml) homemade beef
stock (page 84)

1 large whole onion, peeled (about
the size of a fist)

10 cloves garlic, peeled

1 tablespoon (9 g) powdered
mustard

1 tablespoon (2.5 g) fresh thyme
leaves

1 tablespoon (2.5 g) chopped fresh
sage

1 tablespoon (15 ml) apple cider
vinegar

2 cups (260 g) sliced carrots, 1-inch
(2.5 cm) wide

4 red potatoes, scrubbed and
quartered

2 cups (300 g) peeled and large
diced turnips (about 2 medium)

Preheat the oven to 325ºF (170ºC, or gas mark 3) and move the racks to the bottom of the oven. Rinse the meat and dry thoroughly with a paper towel. Lay the meat on a plate and sprinkle evenly with 1½ teaspoons of the sea salt and 1 teaspoon of the pepper. Drag the meat around the plate to collect any stray seasoning.

In a 6-quart (5.4 L) heavy-bottomed enamel-coated, cast-iron or stainless steel pot over medium-high heat, melt the ghee until glistening. Add the meat to the pan; it will sizzle when it touches the hot ghee. Brown each side for 1½ to 2 minutes. Do not move the meat until ready to turn or the meat will stick to the pan (it will release easily when done). While the meat is searing, wash the used plate. When all sides are brown, remove the meat to rest on the clean plate.

Lower the heat to medium and add the butter and chopped onion to the now-empty pan. Sauté for 5 minutes, stirring occasionally, until softened. Slowly add 1 cup (235 ml) of the broth, scraping browned bits from the bottom of the pan. Add the remaining 4 cups (940 ml) broth, whole onion and garlic, mustard, thyme, sage, apple cider vinegar, and remaining 1½ teaspoons sea salt and ½ teaspoon pepper. Cover and bring to a boil, then turn off the heat, uncover, and add the meat back to the pan. Cover and place the pot in the preheated oven.

Roast for 2 hours, then remove from oven and discard the whole onion. Flip the roast over and add the carrots and

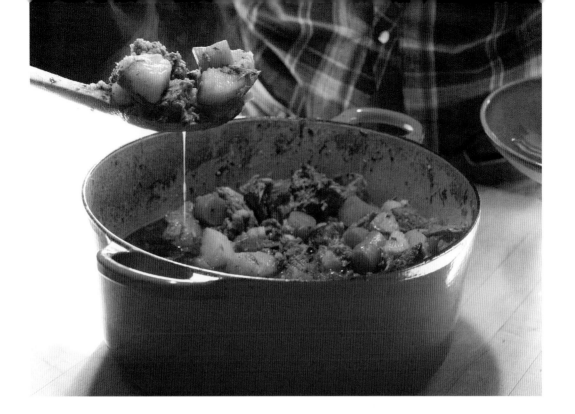

potatoes to the broth. Cover and return the pot to the oven. Roast for 30 minutes, then remove from the oven and add the turnips. Cover again and roast for 30 minutes more. When ready, a fork can quite easily pull apart the roast.

Remove from the oven, uncover, and transfer the roast only to a low-sided ceramic bowl. Replace the lid to the pot of vegetables and set aside.

Shred the meat using two forks; you want medium- and large-size chunks that will ladle fairly easily into a bowl. Carefully slide the shredded meat back into the pot of broth and vegetables. Stir gently to combine then return to the oven, uncovered, for an additional 15 minutes. This will slightly thicken the sauce, finish cooking the vegetables, and allow the meat to be thoroughly seasoned by the broth.

Serve family style or ladle into individual bowls. Remember to add a ladle of broth on top of each individual serving.

YIELD: 10 SERVINGS

Mom used to make this comforting dish with a can of mushroom soup. When filtered through a traditional foods lens, we substitute a simple mushroom gravy, made from bone broth with fresh herbs.

Meatballs & Mushroom Gravy

2 eggs

1 pound (454 g) ground beef

1 pound (454 g) ground pork

1 tablespoon (14 g) minced beef heart, optional

1 cup (160 g) small diced yellow onion, divided

4½ teaspoons (27 g) sea salt, divided

1 teaspoon freshly cracked pepper, divided

2 tablespoons (30 ml) ghee (page 22)

6 tablespoons (84 g) butter, divided

1 pound (454 g) cleaned and destemmed button mushrooms, diced small

1 tablespoon (10 g) minced garlic

2 tablespoons (8 g) chopped fresh flat-leaf parsley

2 tablespoons (6 g) chopped fresh chives

3½ cups (822 ml) homemade beef stock (page 84), divided

½ cup (60 g) fresh-milled, sprouted whole wheat flour (page 55)

2 pounds (908 g) red potatoes

¾ cup (180 ml) milk

YIELD: 4 TO 6 SERVINGS

In large-size mixing bowl, add the eggs and beat with a fork for 30 seconds. Add the beef, pork, beef heart (if using), ½ cup (80 g) of the onion, 1 teaspoon of the sea salt, and ¼ teaspoon of the pepper. Mix carefully with your fingers; do not overmix, as this creates tough meatballs. Using a 2¼-inch (5.7 cm) cookie scoop and/or your hands, shape 16 to 18 meatballs, slightly larger than a golf ball. Place the meatballs on a clean plate.

In a medium-size stockpot over medium-high heat, melt the ghee until glistening. Place half the meatballs into the hot ghee, spacing them out evenly. If the ghee is beginning to brown and sizzle aggressively, turn the heat down to medium. Sauté the meatballs for 2 minutes per side, until nicely browned. When properly browned, the meatballs will turn easily using a spoon, spatula, or tongs. If a meatball will not turn, continue cooking until it does. If it is still sticking after additional cooking, use a kitchen spoon to gently scoop under the meatball and dislodge the meat from the pan. If this happens repeatedly, reduce the heat a bit.

When the meatballs are browned, remove them with tongs to a clean plate. Continue with the second half of the meatballs; no additional ghee will be needed. When finished, add the meatballs to the plate and set aside.

Using the same stockpot (without cleaning) over medium heat, melt 2 tablespoons (28 g) of the butter until foaming. Add the mushrooms and remaining ½ cup (80 g) onion. Using a wooden spoon, scrape the bits of meat from the bottom of the pan as the mushrooms release their moisture. Sauté for 5 minutes, until softened. Add the garlic, parsley, chives,

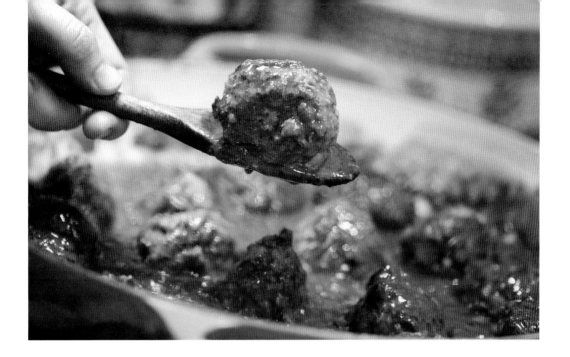

2 teaspoons (12 g) sea salt and ½ teaspoon pepper, and sauté for 2 additional minutes. Add 3 cups (705 ml) of the stock, raise the heat to high, and bring to a boil. Reduce the heat to maintain a rolling simmer.

While the sauce is simmering, in a small-size jar with a lid, combine the remaining ½ cup (120 ml) stock and the flour. Cover and shake very well. Slowly pour the flour mixture into the simmering sauce, whisking constantly. Whisk for 1 minute, while the sauce thickens. Carefully, using tongs, add the meatballs back into the pan. Cover, reduce the heat slightly, and gently simmer for 90 minutes.

While the meatballs are simmering, scrub the potatoes (but do not peel), pare away bad spots, and chop into 1-inch (2.5 cm) chunks. In a medium-size pot with a lid, place the potatoes, 1 teaspoon sea salt, and enough water to cover by 2 inches (5 cm). Cover and set aside.

Forty-five minutes before serving, over high heat, bring the potatoes to a boil. Once boiling, uncover and reduce the heat to medium. Boil gently for 30 minutes, until the potatoes can be pierced easily with a fork, then turn off the heat, drain well in a colander, and return immediately to the hot pot. Add the milk, 3 tablespoons (42 g) of the butter, remaining ½ teaspoon sea salt, and remaining ¼ teaspoon pepper. Return the heat to medium-high and heat until the milk is barely simmering, then remove from the heat. Beat the potatoes slowly with an electric mixer until the butter is melted. The potatoes can be left slightly chunky, if desired. Place in a serving bowl, and top with the remaining 1 tablespoon (14 g) butter, for garnish.

After 90 minutes, taste the gravy and if needed, re-season the sauce. To serve, dollop a mound of potatoes on a plate, top with a couple of meatballs, and smother it all with a big ladle of gravy. Delish!

This pie is similar to shepherd's pie, but the bottom is a tomato-based beef filling while the top is slathered with creamy hominy grits, as opposed to potatoes. Hominy grits are the traditionally treated (page 59) version of polenta. The careful lime treatment results in the creamiest, softest corn and truly makes the dish.

Hominy Pie

FOR HOMINY GRITS:

3 cups (705 ml) homemade chicken
　　stock (page 82)

1 teaspoon sea salt

1 cup (140 g) fresh-milled hominy
　　grits (page 61)

½ cup (50 g) finely grated Parmesan

FOR FILLING:

1 tablespoon (15 ml) ghee (page 22),
　　plus additional for the pan

½ cup (80 g) small diced red onion

1 tablespoon (10 g) minced garlic

1 pound (454 g) ground beef

½ cup (75 g) small diced red bell
　　pepper

1 cup (70 g) thinly sliced cremini
　　mushrooms

2 cups (470 ml) Bone Broth Marinara
　　(page 121)

1 tablespoon (14 g) minced liver

½ cup (60 g) small diced zucchini

½ teaspoon sea salt

½ teaspoon freshly cracked pepper

2 tablespoons (5 g) chopped fresh
　　basil

4 ounces (112 g) fresh whole milk
　　mozzarella, crumbled

TO MAKE THE HOMINY GRITS: In a medium-size pot with tall sides over high heat, bring the stock and sea salt to a boil. Slowly pour in the grits while whisking to prevent lumps. Lower the heat to medium-low and simmer slowly for 30 minutes, whisking every 3 minutes; the grits should produce large, sputtering bubbles. Remove from the heat. Whisk in the Parmesan.

TO MAKE THE FILLING: In a large-size saucepan with tall sides over medium heat, melt the ghee. Add the onion, garlic, and beef, and using a potato masher or wooden spoon, crumble the ground beef for 1 minute. Add the red pepper and mushrooms and sauté for about 12 minutes. Adjust the heat to evaporate liquid.

Add the marinara, liver (if using), zucchini, sea salt, and pepper. Continue to cook over medium-low heat for 5 minutes, stirring occasionally. Remove from the heat. Stir in the basil.

Preheat the oven to 350ºF (180ºC, or gas mark 4). Coat an 8 x 8-inch (20 x 20 cm) glass baking dish lightly with ghee. Spread the beef mixture into the bottom of the pan. Spread the crumbled mozzarella evenly over the top, followed by the grits, using a spatula to spread evenly.

Bake for 50 minutes, uncovered. The grits will brown lightly along the edges and the underlayer of sauce will be bubbling. Let stand for 10 minutes. Serve warm.

YIELD: 4 TO 6 SERVINGS

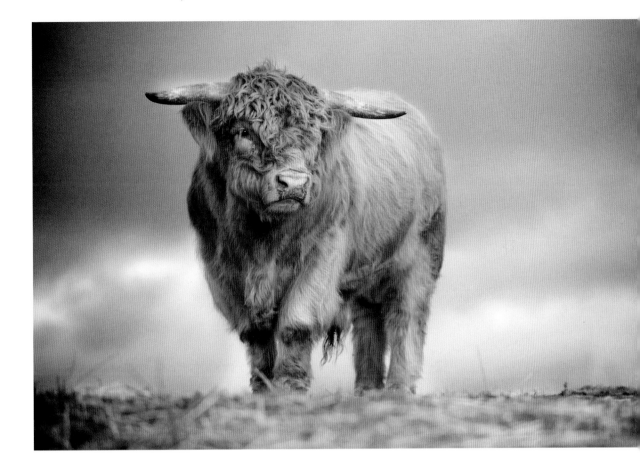

RECIPE NOTES

• Fresh mozzarella is often stored in water. Dry the mozzarella well with a cloth or paper towel before crumbling.

• To coat a pan lightly in ghee, spread room-temperature or melted ghee onto the pan using a folded paper towel.

• If using store-bought sauce, the sauce may be more watery than when using the Bone Broth Marinara. In that case, raise the heat to medium-high after adding the marinara and cook until the sauce is quite thick and not at all watery.

When I make this dish, my kitchen smells like the scent of my childhood. I think it's the smell of grated onion and chopped parsley. Grating onion was my mom's way of hiding it from us when my brother and I were younger. We didn't know that it was only the texture we didn't like! Plus, meatloaf is a delicious place to hide all sorts of things. These days, we hide a bit of minced liver, too. Organ meats are so important for our overall health, yet people often think they don't like them. So we just hide 'em instead!

Mom's Meatloaf

2 eggs

1 pound (454 g) ground beef

1 pound (454 g) ground pork

1 tablespoon (14 g) minced liver, optional

½ cup (25 g) Sourdough Bread Crumbs (page 188)

¼ cup (60 g) plus ⅓ cup (80 g) ketchup (page 174), divided

⅓ cup (55 g) finely grated yellow onion

1 teaspoon fish sauce (see Note)

1 teaspoon minced garlic

2 tablespoons (8 g) chopped fresh flat-leaf parsley

1 teaspoon sea salt

⅛ teaspoon pepper

2 slices uncooked bacon, roughly chopped

YIELD: 6 TO 8 SERVINGS

Preheat the oven to 350°F (180°C, or gas mark 4). Have ready a glass or ceramic loaf pan (no need to grease the pan).

Into a medium-size bowl, crack the eggs and beat with a fork for 30 seconds. Add the beef, pork, liver (if using), bread crumbs, ¼ cup (60 g) ketchup, onion, fish sauce, garlic, parsley, sea salt, and pepper. Use your fingers to gently mix together for approximately 30 seconds. Avoid overmixing as this toughens the meat.

Gently press the mixture evenly into the pan. Spread the remaining ⅓ cup (80 g) ketchup and chopped bacon over the top of the meat.

Bake for 1 hour and 20 minutes. When done, the loaf will pull away slightly from the sides of the pan, and the topping will be somewhat crispy and browned. Allow the meatloaf to rest for 5 minutes before slicing into 1-inch (2.5 cm) pieces. Serve warm.

RECIPE NOTE

This recipe originally used Worcestershire sauce instead of naturally fermented fish sauce, which we call for here. Store-bought Worcestershire sauce contains soy sauce, most likely of low quality and minimally fermented, and should therefore be avoided as mentioned on page 50. Soy should only be eaten in its traditionally fermented state. However, if unable to source a high-quality Worcestershire sauce, fermented fish sauce serves as a delicious and nutritious substitute.

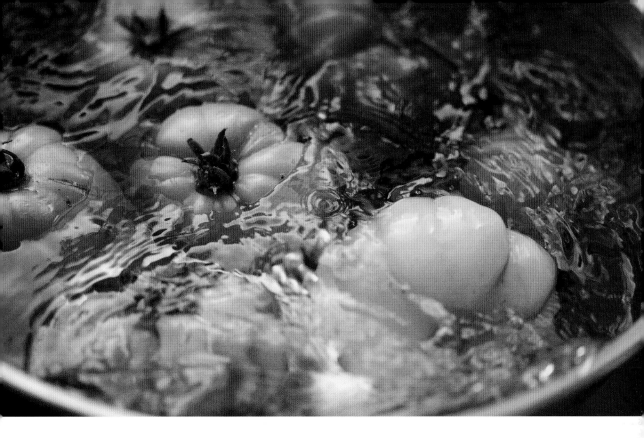

CHAPTER 10

SEASONAL SIDES

SIDE DISHES ARE OFTEN OUR FAVORITE PART OF A MEAL and even guide the split decision of a main course at a restaurant. They capture and translate the colors and textures of each season. Eating seasonally parades earth's best offerings at their peak. A red, juicy watermelon says summertime better than any spoken word, while proud asparagus stands tall with a bold salute to spring.

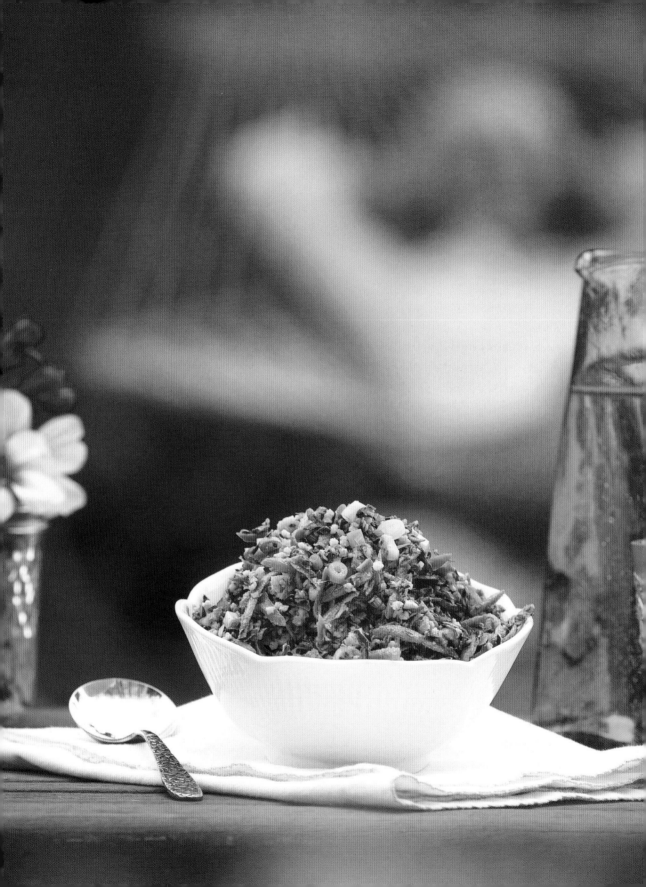

This recipe used to be called Whole Grain and Crisp Vegetable Slaw—snooze. During the photo shoot, we commented on how the brightly colored carrots, cabbage, and scallions almost made the dish look like confetti! Bye-bye, boring name (though it's still delicious no matter what you call it)!

Confetti Slaw

FOR SALAD:

1½ cups (195 g) shredded carrot

1½ cups (105 g) shredded red
    cabbage

⅓ cup (35 g) sliced scallion, both
    white and green parts

⅓ cup (37 g) roughly chopped
    crunchy walnuts (page 49)

⅓ cup (30 g) diced fennel

¼ cup (16 g) chopped fresh flat-leaf
    parsley

¾ cup (140 g) cooked millet
    (page 53)

FOR DRESSING:

5 tablespoons (75 ml) unrefined
    walnut oil

2 tablespoons (30 ml) apple cider
    vinegar

2 teaspoons Dijon mustard

2 teaspoons raw honey

½ teaspoon sea salt

¼ teaspoon freshly cracked pepper

YIELD: 4 TO 6 SERVINGS

TO MAKE THE SALAD: In a medium-size bowl, combine the salad ingredients. Toss with a fork and set aside.

TO MAKE THE DRESSING: In a small-size bowl, combine the dressing ingredients, whisking until well combined.

Right before serving, pour the dressing over the salad and toss with a fork.

Amid the first breaths of spring, out of some unsuspecting patch of ground, incredibly sturdy green shoots of asparagus come poking up. In this dish, the spears are blanched to enhance their bright green color, then cooled, drizzled with a simple marinade, and served cold, making it a perfect party dish.

Chilled Sweet 'n Sour Asparagus

Inspired by Karen Wilmer

1½ pounds (680 g) asparagus

2 cups (470 ml) water

1 teaspoon sea salt

2 tablespoons (30 ml) unrefined sesame oil

¼ cup (60 ml) apple cider vinegar

¼ cup (60 ml) Nama shoyu

¼ cup (80 g) raw honey

¾ cup (83 g) crunchy pecans (page 49), coarsely broken

YIELD: 4 SERVINGS

RECIPE NOTE

Nama shoyu is an unpasteurized raw soy sauce with beneficial organisms intact. If Nama shoyu cannot be found, try shoyu or tamari, which are pasteurized, but still fermented. For those who cannot tolerate soy in any form, try coconut aminos (page 217).

Trim 1 to 2 inches (2.5 to 5 cm) from the bottom of the asparagus spears to remove the tough portion of the stalk.

In a large-size saucepan with tall sides, combine the water and sea salt. Over high heat, bring to a boil covered. As soon as the water is boiling, add the asparagus, cover, and turn the heat down to medium-high for 2 minutes. Fill a large-size bowl with ice water.

After the 2-minute blanch, using tongs, quickly transfer the asparagus to the bowl of ice water to stop the cooking process. After 2 minutes in ice water, use tongs to carefully transfer the asparagus to a colander and drain thoroughly.

Combine the sesame oil, apple cider vinegar, Nama shoyu, and honey. Whisk vigorously to combine.

Place asparagus in a glass dish (with a cover) and pour the dressing over the top. Cover and refrigerate for 2 to 6 hours.

To serve, use tongs to transfer asparagus to a serving platter, then pour the remaining dressing back over the top. Garnish with the pecan pieces and serve cold.

Color abounds with this dish. The chives add a fresh bright pop to the deep dark purple of the beets—we think you'll agree it's a beautiful combination! This side is a wonderful addition to a couple of fried pastured eggs on a Saturday morning.

Caramelized Beets with Fresh Chives

1½ pounds beets, peeled and thinly sliced

2 tablespoons (30 ml) bacon fat (page 33)

⅛ teaspoon sea salt

⅛ teaspoon fresh cracked pepper

2 tablespoons (6 g) chopped fresh chives

YIELD: 4 SERVINGS

In large skillet (with a lid) over medium heat, melt bacon fat. Once melted, add sliced beets and toss to coat. Reduce heat to low, cover, and gently cook for 25 minutes, stirring occasionally.

After 25 minutes, remove the lid and increase the heat to medium. Sauté for an additional 5 minutes, without stirring, to finish caramelizing.

After five minutes, remove from the heat. Add sea salt, pepper, and chives. Toss to combine and serve warm.

RECIPE NOTE

Save the beet greens for another use, such as in a soup or salad, or sautéed with butter and garlic.

Have you ever seen potatoes grow? First, you let them sprout in the greenhouse before planting them in soil prepared with a bit of compost. As they grow, the gardener mounds the dirt up around the plant so the area becomes a bit of a hill. As our vegetable garden manager at Apricot Lane says, "You can't mess up a potato."

Picnic Potato Salad

4 eggs

2 pounds (908 g) red potatoes, scrubbed, with bad spots removed

2 teaspoons (12 g) sea salt, divided

⅔ cup (150 g) Simply Mayonnaise (page 178)

2 tablespoons (28 g) sour cream

¼ teaspoon freshly cracked black pepper

2 tablespoons (8 g) fresh parsley

2 tablespoons (6 g) fresh chives

2 tablespoons (30 g) Fermented Sweet Pickle Relish (page 173), drained well

2 tablespoons (40 g) raw honey

1 teaspoon apple cider vinegar

½ cup (80 g) small diced sweet onion

¼ cup (25 g) diagonally sliced scallion, both white and green parts

Paprika, for garnish

YIELD: 8 SERVINGS

Place the eggs in a small-size pot with tall sides and fill with enough water to cover by 2 inches (5 cm). In a medium-size pot, place the potatoes and 1 teaspoon sea salt and fill with enough water to cover the potatoes by 2 inches (5 cm). Cover both pots and bring to a boil over high heat. Once boiling, uncover. Boil the eggs for 10 minutes. Boil the potatoes for approximately 15 minutes, or until just fork tender.

While the eggs and potatoes are cooking, in a small-size bowl, combine the remaining 1 teaspoon sea salt, mayonnaise, sour cream, pepper, parsley, chives, relish, honey, and vinegar.

When the eggs finish cooking, remove and drain. Refill the pot with cold water and allow the eggs to cool to the touch. When the potatoes finish cooking, drain in a colander and set aside to cool slightly.

Peel the eggs and roughly chop into ¼-inch (6 mm) pieces. Place in a large-size bowl. Chop the potatoes into ½-inch (1.3 cm) pieces (do not peel), carefully avoiding mashing. Add the potatoes to the bowl with the eggs, followed by the sweet onion and scallion.

Pour the mayonnaise mixture over the warm potato mixture and gently fold together with a spatula.

Place the mixture into a serving bowl. Chill overnight or for several hours and serve cold. If needed, at serving time, "refresh" by folding a bit more mayo into the salad and sprinkle with paprika, for garnish.

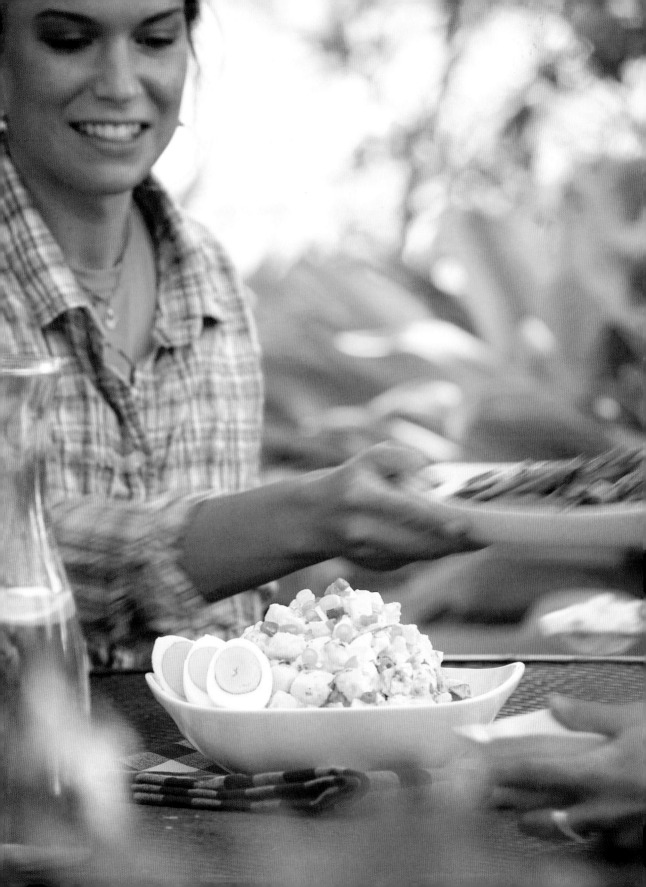

I got married on the summer solstice with a reception at an inspired restaurant in Berlin, Maryland, called Solstice (the name was a total coincidence). It was a beautiful day, filled with delicious farm-to-table food. There were lots of fun things about that day, but if you asked Mom for her favorite, she'd tell you about the succotash. I don't know how they did it, but this is our version of the original. Note that there is a minimum of 12 hours of advance prep time.

Sufferin' Succotash

2 cups (340 g) fresh or frozen lima
   beans (no need to defrost)
2 tablespoons (30 ml) whey (page 40)
3 ounces (84 g) medium diced
   pancetta
3 tablespoons (42 g) butter, divided
1 cup (100 g) diagonally sliced
   scallion, both white and
   green parts
¼ cup (38 g) small diced red bell
   pepper
½ cup (75 g) halved cherry tomatoes
2 cups (470 ml) water
1 teaspoon sea salt, divided
2½ cups (375 g) fresh corn cut off
   the cob
½ cup (75 g) fresh corn grated off
   the cob
1½ cups (355 ml) cream
¼ teaspoon white pepper, or to taste
1 teaspoon chopped flat-leaf parsley,
   for garnish

YIELD: 4 TO 6 SERVINGS

In a small-size saucepan, combine the lima beans, whey, and enough water to generously cover. Cover the pot and set aside in a warm spot for 12 to 24 hours. Drain and rinse well before continuing with the recipe.

In a small-size nonstick sauté pan over medium heat, add the pancetta and sauté uncovered until browned and crispy, approximately 10 minutes. Using a slotted spoon, remove from the pan and place on a plate covered with a paper towel. Leave the pancetta renderings in the pan and add 1 table-spoon (14 g) of the butter.

Raise the heat to medium and when the butter is melted, add the scallion, red pepper, and tomatoes. Sauté for 3 to 4 min-utes, stirring frequently, until lightly softened. Remove from the heat and set aside.

In a medium-size saucepan with a lid, combine the lima beans, water, and ½ teaspoon sea salt. With the saucepan covered and over high heat, bring the liquid to a boil. Lower the heat to medium and maintain a rolling simmer, covered, for 12 min-utes. Add the cut corn, re-cover, and cook for 3 more minutes. Turn off the heat.

In a colander, quickly drain the cut corn and lima beans and return them to the hot pot. Add the remaining 2 tablespoons (28 g) butter, cover, and let stand while the butter melts. Add the grated corn, cream, remaining ½ teaspoon sea salt, and pepper.

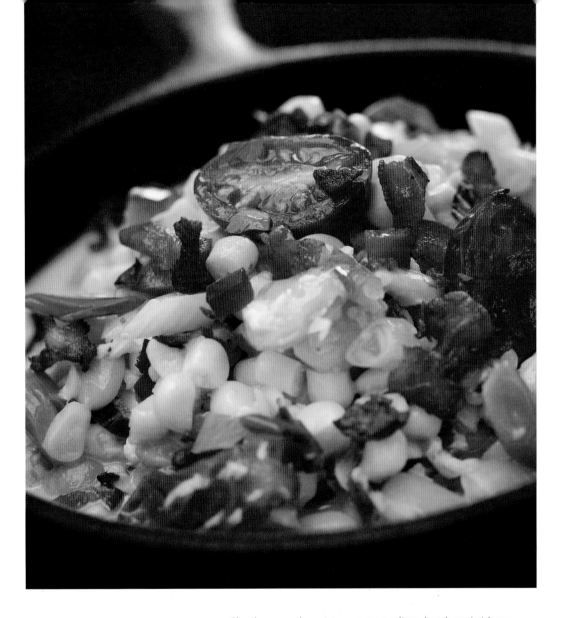

Slowly warm the mixture over medium-low heat (without boiling), stirring frequently. When heated through, add the pancetta and vegetable sauté. Continue stirring and warming until fully heated. Taste and re-season with sea salt and pepper, if necessary.

Transfer to a serving dish and sprinkle with the parsley. Serve warm.

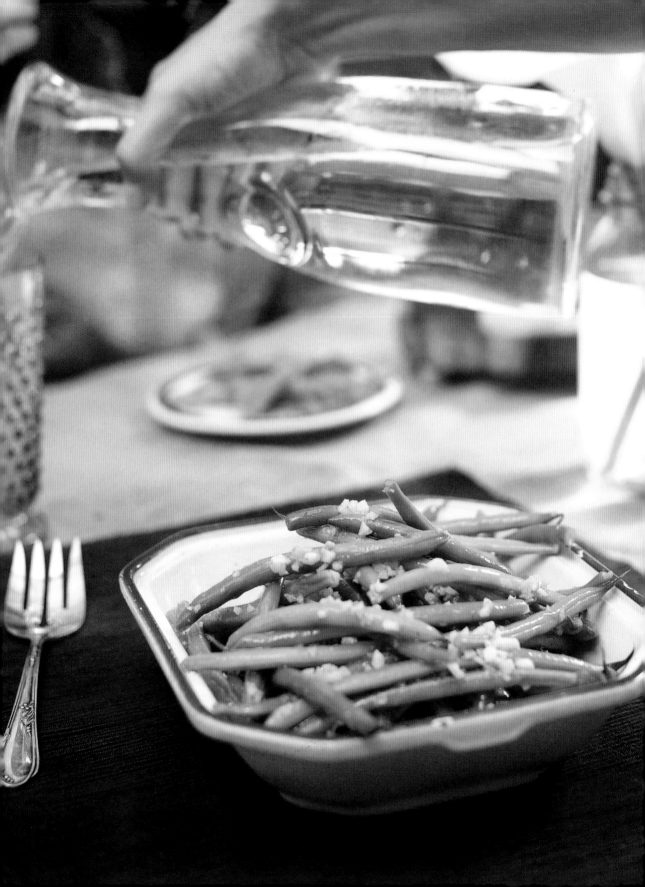

For this simple and crowd-pleasing recipe, the blanching and shocking method is used. This technique enables you to precook the vegetables to the desired crispness before arresting the cooking process with ice-cold water. In the last-minute rush to get dinner on the table, the veggies are simply reheated and served! Try it once and you'll understand why restaurants do this all the time.

Garden Green Beans with Garlic & Olive Oil

10 cups (2350 ml) water

2 tablespoons (36 g) plus
   ¾ teaspoon sea salt, divided

1 pound (454 g) fresh green beans

3 tablespoons (45 ml) extra-virgin
   olive oil

5 cloves garlic, minced

¼ teaspoon freshly cracked pepper

YIELD: 4 SERVINGS

In a large-size pot with a lid, bring the water and 2 tablespoons (36 g) of the sea salt to a boil, covered.

Snap or cut the stem ends off of the beans. When the water comes to a boil, add the beans, return to a boil, and boil for 6 minutes. Meanwhile, fill a large-size bowl with ice water. After 6 minutes, scoop the beans out of the boiling water and into the ice water bath using a slotted spoon. Allow the beans to chill for 2 minutes, then strain and set aside.

Right before serving, heat the olive oil in a large-size sauté pan over medium heat for 1 minute. Add the garlic and sauté for 30 seconds. Add the beans, remaining ¾ teaspoon sea salt, and the pepper to the pan. Toss with tongs for 3 minutes, until heated through. Serve immediately.

Apricot Lane has mobile chicken coops that move pasture to pasture after the sheep are herded to new grass. The chickens pile out of their coop in the morning, returning unprompted at dusk, just in time for us to close it up. The effort to keep chickens on a patch of fresh green grass does not go unreturned. Those chickens produce eggs with a color of orange that is unable to be faked. It's their "thank you" back to the farmer.

Creamy Deviled Eggs

8 eggs

3 tablespoons (42 g) Simply Mayonnaise (page 178)

1 tablespoon (14 g) Yogurt Cream Cheese (page 40)

2 tablespoons (30 g) Sweet Pickle Relish (page 173)

⅛ teaspoon sea salt

⅛ teaspoon white pepper

1 teaspoon Dijon mustard

2 teaspoons (2 g) chopped fresh chives

1 teaspoon honey

Paprika, for garnish

YIELD: 8 SERVINGS

Place the eggs in a medium-size pot and add enough water to cover by 2 inches (5 cm). Cover the pot and bring to a boil over high heat. Once boiling, remove the lid and boil for 10 minutes. If necessary, lower the heat to medium-high to keep the water from spilling over. After 10 minutes, turn off the heat and drain. Allow the eggs to cool to the touch before peeling.

Meanwhile, in a small-size bowl, combine the mayonnaise, cream cheese, relish, sea salt, pepper, mustard, chives, and honey. Whisk to combine.

Once the eggs are cooled, peel and cut in half lengthwise. Carefully remove the yolk of each egg half and place in a small-size flat-bottomed bowl. Mash the yolks well with a potato masher. Add the mayonnaise mixture to the mashed yolks. Stir well with a spoon to combine. Taste, adding additional sea salt as desired.

Using a teaspoon, carefully fill the cavity of each egg with the yolk mixture. Gently sprinkle the top of each with a dash of paprika. Cover and refrigerate for several hours or overnight before serving.

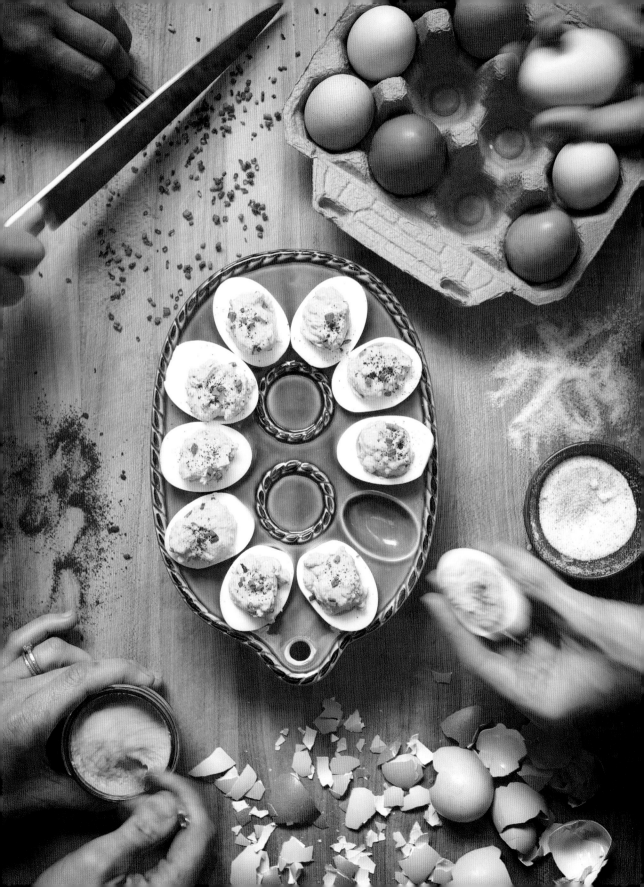

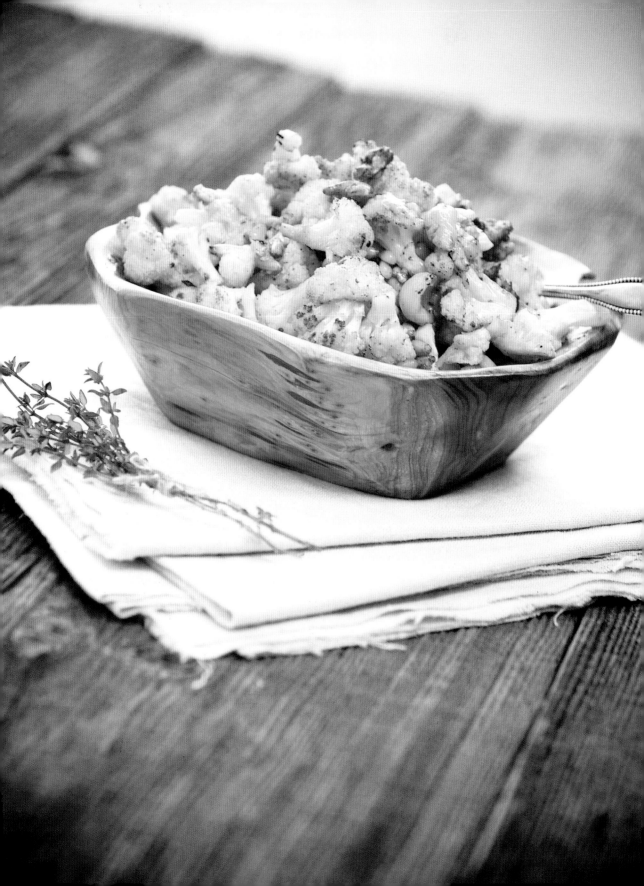

Cooking feels the best to me when it has an element of "throwing it all together." I love to feel the freedom of tossing things into a dish, popping it in the oven, and coming out the other side with a roasted, delicious pile of good food. This dish is a perfect example. Case in point: If you can't find golden raisins, regular raisins or currants will work just fine.

Roasted Cauliflower with Pine Nuts & Parmesan

¼ cup (60 ml) bacon fat (page 33)

6 cloves garlic, smashed but whole

5 cups (500 g) bite-size cauliflower florets (about 1 large head)

⅓ cup (45 g) pine nuts

¼ teaspoon sea salt

½ teaspoon freshly cracked pepper

3 whole fresh thyme sprigs

¼ cup (25 g) freshly grated Parmesan, optional

⅓ cup (50 g) golden raisins

YIELD: 4 SERVINGS

Preheat the oven to 425°F (220°C, or gas mark 7). Melt the fat in a small-size pot over medium heat.

In a 9 x 13-inch (23 x 33 cm) glass baking dish, combine the smashed garlic, cauliflower, and pine nuts. Drizzle the melted renderings over the cauliflower mixture, and sprinkle the sea salt and pepper over the top. Toss well with a spatula until the cauliflower is evenly coated. Place the thyme sprigs on top.

Bake for 25 minutes, then turn with a spatula, and sprinkle the Parmesan on top, if desired. Bake for 15 minutes more, until the edges of the cauliflower have caramelized and the nuts are nicely browned.

Place the pan on a cooling rack and remove the thyme stems. Add the raisins and toss well. Serve warm.

RECIPE NOTE

Bring the cauliflower to room temperature before preparation and dry thoroughly after rinsing. The bacon fat will seize if the cauliflower is cold, and extra moisture will prevent the dish from browning.

Taking the time to properly prepare beans makes such a difference for the after-party. No more bellyaches. No more open windows. And think about it, if your belly is that upset, you can't possibly be digesting properly. Weak digestion means that your body is not receiving the proper building blocks for energy and vitality!

Meaty Baked Beans

8 ounces (225 g) bacon, roughly chopped

1 tablespoon (15 ml) reserved bacon drippings

1¼ cups (200 g) small diced yellow onion

1 pound (454 g) ground beef

1 tablespoon (14 g) chicken liver, optional

1 tablespoon (14 g) butter

1 cup (240 g) ketchup (page 174)

⅓ cup (105 g) raw honey

1 tablespoon (15 ml) maple syrup

1 teaspoon prepared yellow mustard (page 177)

3 cups (510 g) cooked Great Northern beans (page 52), plus ½ cup (120 ml) reserved bean cooking liquid

YIELD: 6 TO 8 SERVINGS

RECIPE NOTE

The beans recipe on page 52 must be doubled for this dish.

Preheat the oven to 350ºF (180ºC, or gas mark 4). In a large-size skillet over medium-high heat, cook the bacon until crisp, stirring occasionally, approximately 10 minutes. Remove with a slotted spoon and drain on a paper towel–lined plate. Pour the renderings into a clean glass jar to cool. Measure 1 tablespoon (15 ml) bacon drippings back into the same pan. Over medium-high heat, add the onion and sauté for approximately 5 minutes, stirring frequently, until softened. Using a slotted spoon, remove the onion and place on the same plate as the cooked bacon (paper towel removed).

Into the same pan over medium-high heat, add the ground beef and sauté until well browned, approximately 8 minutes, occasionally breaking up the meat with a wooden spoon or the tip of a spatula. If the meat begins to stick, lower the heat to medium. When the meat is browned, remove from the heat and add the sautéed onion, bacon, and liver (if using) to the pan. Stir to combine. Bury the butter in the warm mixture and set aside while the butter melts.

In the bottom of a 2-quart (2 L) baking dish, mix the ketchup, honey, maple syrup, and yellow mustard. Stir well. Add the beans and their cooking liquid and the meat mixture. Stir well once more.

Bake, covered, for 25 minutes, then 20 minutes longer either covered or uncovered. If you prefer a thicker consistency, like our family, cook uncovered. If you prefer a thinner sauce with your beans, cook covered. Either way, bake an additional 20 minutes and serve warm.

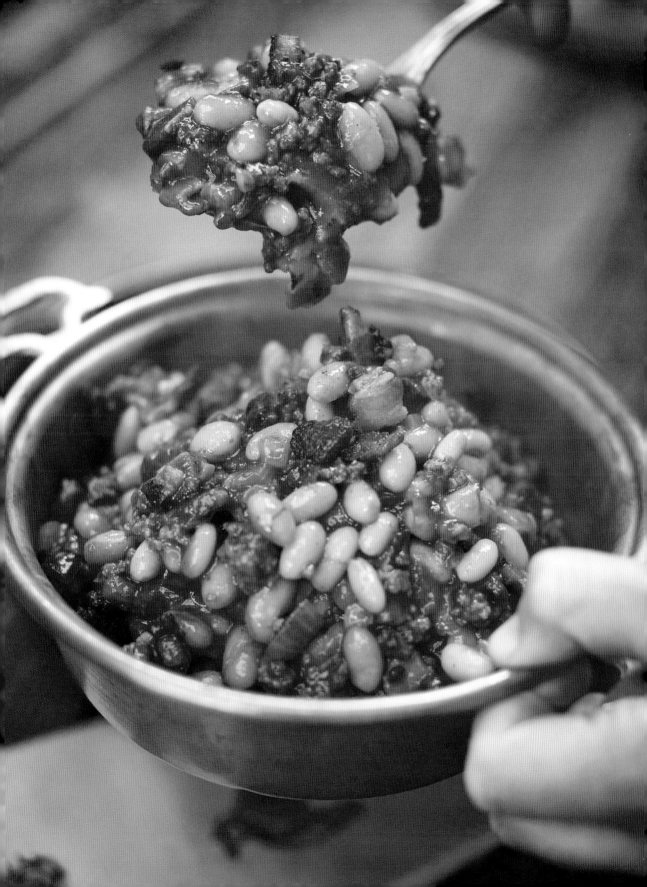

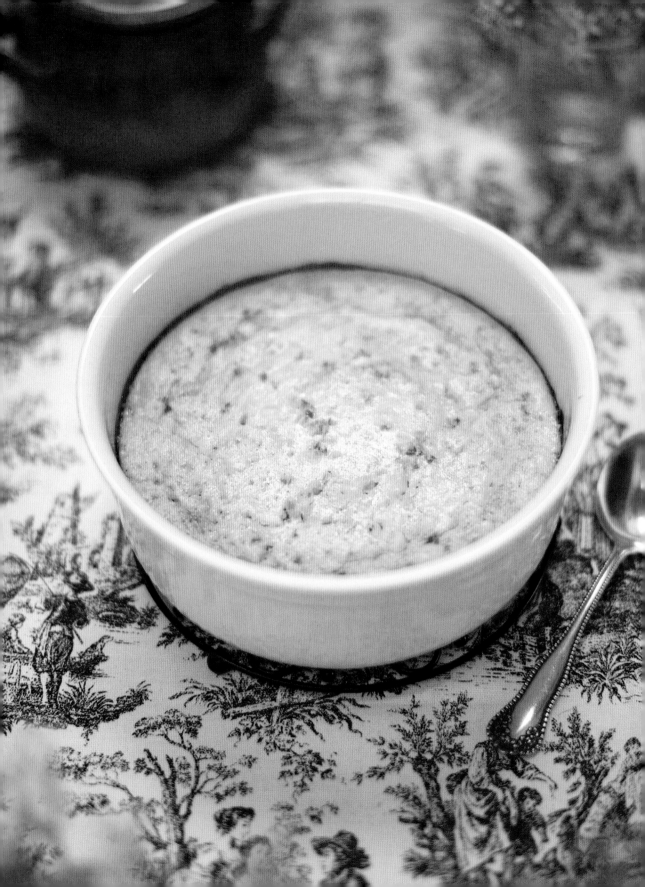

The sound, smell, and feel of walking through dense rows of corn is such a welcome hug of summertime. This dish is a perfect complement to our Sweet Ham Loaf (page 138). Even though fresh is best, frozen corn (from summer's bounty) can certainly be used. Simply pulse ½ cup (65 g) corn in the food processor to substitute for the grated corn.

Fresh Corn Pudding

½ cup (65 g) fresh corn grated off the cob (about 2 medium ears)

1½ cups (195 g) fresh corn cut off the cob (about 3 medium ears)

5 tablespoons (40 g) fresh-milled, sprouted whole wheat pastry flour (page 55)

2 tablespoons (30 ml) maple syrup

1 tablespoon (9 g) seeded and finely chopped jalapeño pepper

½ teaspoon sea salt

¼ teaspoon freshly cracked pepper

4 tablespoons (56 g) butter, melted

4 eggs

1 cup (235 ml) plain kefir (page 42)

YIELD: 4 TO 6 SERVINGS

Preheat the oven to 350ºF (180ºC, or gas mark 4). Have ready a 2-quart (2 L) baking dish.

In a medium-size bowl, combine the corn (grated and whole), flour, maple syrup, jalapeño, sea salt, pepper, and melted butter. Stir well with a spoon to combine.

In a small-size bowl, combine the eggs and kefir, whisking until well combined. Add to the corn mixture and stir until well combined. Pour into the ungreased baking dish.

Bake for 50 minutes to 1 hour, until the pudding rises up the sides of the baking dish and the top turns a delicious golden brown.

RECIPE NOTE

Using a box grater to grate the corn releases the milk from each broken kernel. Note that the amount of corn needed varies depending on the size of the ears. The corn must be thoroughly cleaned of silk and patted dry before grating.

I believe John married me because he had my mom's brussels sprouts at our holiday meals. 'Nuff said.

Brussels Sprouts with Onions and Crispy Bacon

1 pound (454 g) small brussels sprouts, trimmed and halved lengthwise

1½ cups (355 ml) homemade chicken stock (page 82)

1¼ teaspoons sea salt, divided

5 strips bacon, roughly chopped

1½ cups (240 g) thinly sliced yellow onion

3 tablespoons (42 g) butter

½ teaspoon freshly cracked pepper

YIELD: 4 TO 6 SERVINGS

Combine the brussels sprouts, chicken stock, and 1 teaspoon of the sea salt in a 2-quart (1.8 L) pot with a lid. Set aside.

In an extra-large-size nonstick sauté pan over medium heat, cook the bacon until crisp, about 10 minutes. Remove with a slotted spoon and drain on a paper towel–lined plate. Set aside.

In the same pan with the hot bacon drippings, cook the onion over medium-high heat until browned and tender, 6 to 8 minutes. Turn off the heat and set aside.

Over high heat, bring the salted sprouts to a boil. Lower the heat to medium-high and cook for 8 minutes, until fork tender (avoid overcooking sprouts to help retain their shape). Remove from the heat and drain well in a colander, then return to the hot pot. Add the butter, remaining ¼ teaspoon sea salt, and freshly cracked pepper. Cover and allow the butter to melt. Uncover and stir to generously cover the cut side of every sprout with the melted butter.

Heat a large-size cast-iron skillet over low heat and arrange as many sprouts as possible in the pan with the cut side down. Once the sprouts are arranged, raise the heat to medium. Sauté for 5 minutes, without stirring, or until the sprouts are nicely browned. More butter can be added if needed. It may be necessary to brown the sprouts in 2 separate batches to fit. Once nicely browned, turn off the heat.

When ready to serve, warm the caramelized onions slightly and spoon over the browned sprouts, stirring carefully to combine. Sprinkle the crispy bacon over the top and serve immediately.

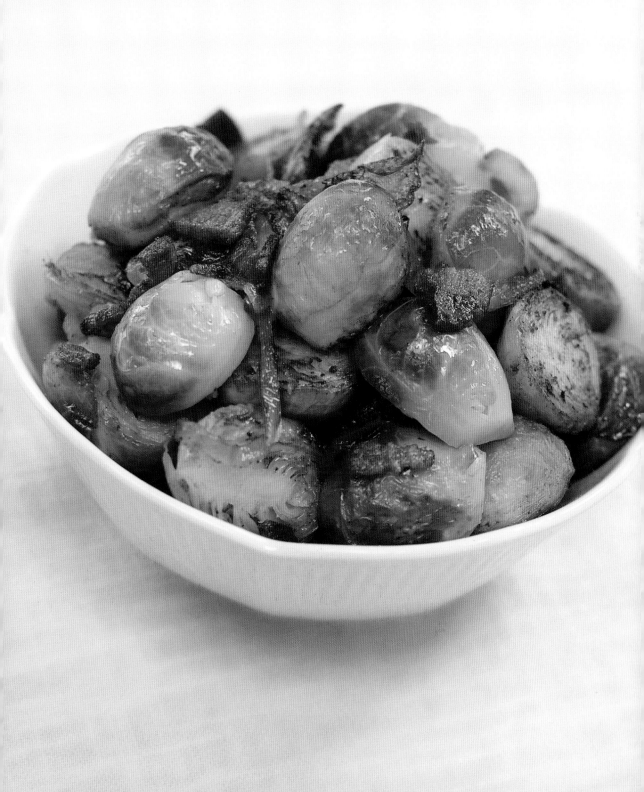

Repeat after me: "Vegetables are good when they are in season." Tomatoes in summer, asparagus in spring, acorn squash in early fall and through the winter—it makes a huge difference in taste. Therefore, don't even try this dish in the spring! The key here is a great, in-season squash.

Baked Acorn Squash with Kale & Pancetta Stuffing

FOR SQUASH:

2 small acorn squash (1 to 1½ pounds [454 to 680 g] each)

12 cloves garlic, peeled

1 cup (235 ml) homemade chicken stock (page 82)

10 whole fresh sage leaves

½ teaspoon sea salt

12 whole black peppercorns

½ teaspoon whole fennel seeds

FOR STUFFING:

½-pound (225 g) chunk pancetta, diced small

⅓ cup (80 ml) reserved pancetta fat

2 cups (300 g) small diced turnip

2 cups (320 g) small diced sweet onion

2 large cloves garlic, thinly sliced

¼ teaspoon crushed red pepper flakes

10 cups (670 g) packed, destemmed, and roughly chopped kale (about 2 bunches)

¼ teaspoon sea salt

2 tablespoons (30 ml) balsamic vinegar

TO MAKE THE SQUASH: Preheat the oven to 350ºF (180ºC, or gas mark 4). Have ready a 9 x 13-inch (23 x 33 cm) glass baking dish.

Cut each squash in half lengthwise from end to end and scoop out the seeds. Do NOT pierce the skin of the squash. Simply place the squash, cut-side down, in the bottom of the glass dish, trapping 1 clove of garlic under each piece of squash. To the surrounding dish, add the stock, remaining 8 garlic cloves, sage, sea salt, peppercorns, and fennel. Bake for 30 to 45 minutes, until the squash can be pierced easily with a fork.

TO MAKE THE STUFFING: In a large-size sauté pan over medium heat, brown the pancetta until crispy and the fat has melted away, stirring frequently. With a slotted spoon, transfer bits of pancetta to a paper towel–lined plate. Set aside. Pour the hot fat into a glass measuring cup, to control the amount used in the next step.

Pour ⅓ cup (80 ml) hot pancetta fat back into the pan, and over medium heat, sauté the turnips for 5 minutes. Add the onion and continue to sauté over medium heat for an additional 5 minutes, stirring frequently. Add the garlic and red pepper flakes, and sauté 1 additional minute, stirring constantly. Lower the heat to medium-low, add the kale, cover, and cook for 3 minutes. Then remove the lid, add the sea salt, balsamic vinegar, and reserved pancetta. Using tongs, toss the mixture until thoroughly combined.

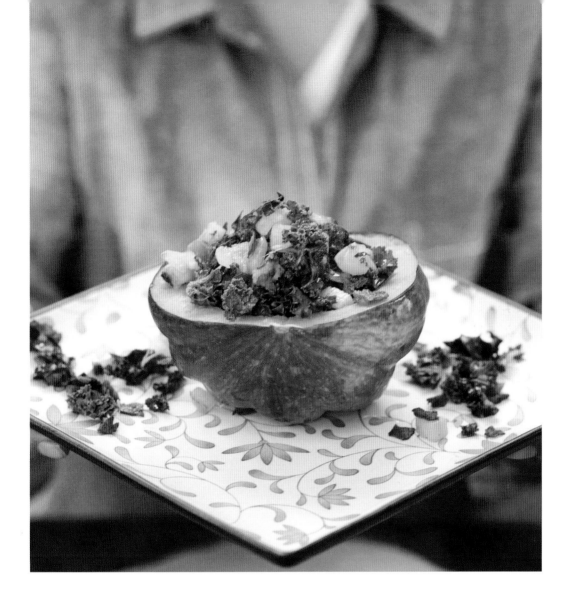

Once fork tender, remove the squash from the oven. Carefully turn the squash cut side up into individual serving dishes. Remove any herbs that may have clung to the squash meat. Liberally sprinkle sea salt and pepper over each squash, then fill each cavity with a liberal cup of kale mixture. Serve warm.

YIELD: 4 SERVINGS, 1 HALF SQUASH AND 1 CUP STUFFING EACH

RECIPE NOTES

• The rendered pancetta fat may not supply a full ⅓ cup (80 ml). If this is the case, simply add enough melted butter to produce the needed amount.

• A salad spinner works nicely here to remove unwanted moisture from the freshly washed kale.

seasonal sides

This recipe is a "choose-your-own-ending" recipe. Containing both a sweet (holiday) topping and a less sweet (everyday) topping, it is designed to suit your year-round needs. Sweet potatoes, both the white and orange-fleshed varieties, and yams all work well in this dish.

The Reversible Sweet Potato Casserole

FOR CASSEROLE:

2 pounds (908 g) sweet potatoes, peeled and chopped into 2-inch (5 cm) pieces

½ cup (112 g) butter, melted

½ cup (112 g) sour cream

1 teaspoon vanilla extract

1 teaspoon sea salt

2 eggs, beaten

FOR EVERYDAY TOPPING:

1 cup (150 g) crunchy pecan halves (page 49)

1 cup (150 g) crunchy walnuts (page 49)

¼ teaspoon sea salt

½ cup (75 g) roughly chopped dried white figs (also known as Calimyrna)

2 tablespoons (28 g) butter, melted

TO MAKE THE CASSEROLE: In a medium-size pot, add the sweet potatoes and enough water to cover by 2 inches (5 cm). Bring to a boil. Lower the heat to medium and maintain a rolling simmer for 10 minutes, or until the potatoes are fork tender.

Meanwhile, preheat the oven to 350ºF (180ºC, or gas mark 4) and butter an 8 x 8 glass baking dish.

Once the potatoes are tender, drain and place in a large-size bowl. Cool for 5 minutes. Using a hand mixer, beat on low speed to mash. Add the butter, sour cream, vanilla, and sea salt and beat on medium speed to combine. Add the eggs and beat again to combine.

Spread the mixture evenly into the prepared dish and bake for 30 minutes. Choose one of the two toppings below and follow the corresponding instructions.

TO MAKE THE EVERYDAY TOPPING: While the casserole is baking, in the bowl of a food processor, combine the pecans, walnuts, and sea salt. Pulse 20 times; the nuts should be in a uniform crumble, but not a paste. Pour into a medium-size bowl and set aside.

Without rinsing the processor bowl, add the figs. Pulse 10 to 50 times, depending on the dryness of the figs. Extremely dry figs may take about 50 pulses to result in a uniform crumble while softer figs may take only 10 pulses.

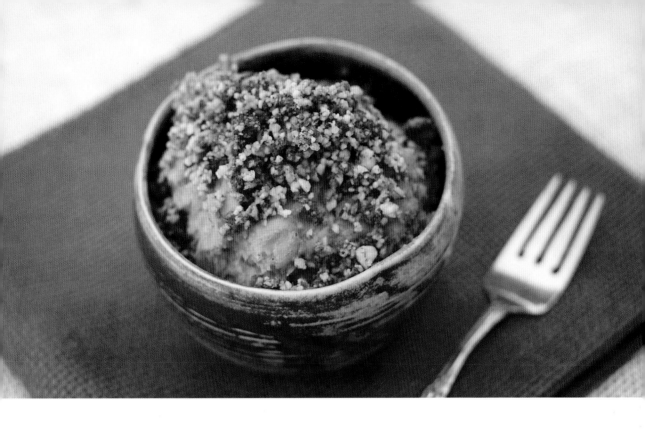

FOR HOLIDAY TOPPING:

⅓ cup (40 g) fresh-milled, sprouted whole wheat pastry flour (page 55)

⅓ cup (67 g) Sucanat (page 64)

1½ cups (225 g) chopped crunchy pecans (page 49)

¼ teaspoon sea salt

1 teaspoon cinnamon

½ cup (112 g) butter, melted

YIELD: 4 TO 6 SERVINGS

Once the figs are adequately chopped, add the nuts back to the processor and pulse the combined mixture 5 times, bringing the nuts and figs into a uniform crumble. Return the mixture to the medium-size bowl and drizzle in the melted butter. Toss with a spatula until combined. The mixture will be crumbly and light.

After the casserole has baked for 30 minutes, remove from the oven and crumble the topping over the casserole. Return to the oven for 15 minutes, or until the topping is lightly browned. Cool for 5 minutes and serve.

TO MAKE THE HOLIDAY TOPPING: While the casserole is baking, combine the flour, Sucanat, pecans, sea salt, and cinnamon in a small-size bowl. Drizzle in the melted butter and mix well by hand. After the casserole has baked for 30 minutes, remove from the oven and crumble the topping over the casserole. Return to the oven for 15 minutes, or until the topping is puffed and lightly browned. Cool 5 minutes and serve.

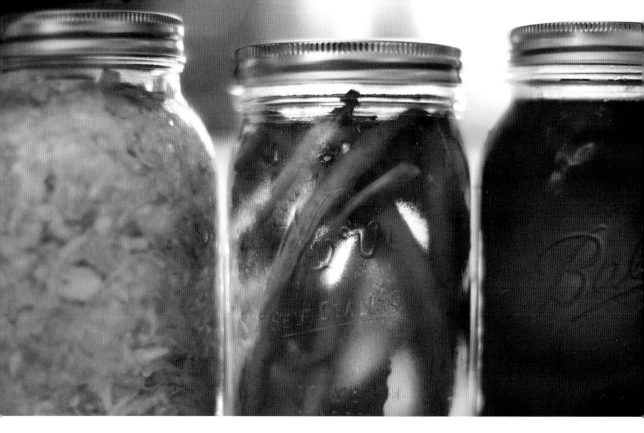

CHAPTER 11

FERMENTED FIXIN'S

MAKING CONDIMENTS AT HOME is a sure-fire way to make you feel fancy. As with store-bought salad dressings, commercial condiments are filled with unhealthy additives, refined oils, sugar, and corn syrup. Compare this to traditional cultures, which relied on basic whole ingredients and fermentation in their condiments, thus increasing digestion and the assimilation of the nutrients in the food. A simple meal of grass-fed hot dogs becomes extra special and nutrient-dense when accompanied by your own homemade fixin's!

Traditionally, the purpose of serving condiments with meals was to aid digestion. Offering fermented condiments not only enhances taste but also provides probiotic cultures, produced during the fermentation process, which help us digest our food. Not only does our modern diet lack fermented condiments, but also many store-bought fixin's contain refined cane sugar, which is known to disrupt, rather than aid, digestion.

Fermented Sweet Pickle Relish

½ cup (80 g) medium diced sweet onion

1 teaspoon minced garlic

2½ cups (300 g) seeded and large diced English cucumber

1 teaspoon sea salt

1 teaspoon celery seed

½ teaspoon mustard seed

3 tablespoons (60 g) raw honey

3 tablespoons (45 ml) traditionally fermented green cabbage sauerkraut juice (see Resources, page 216)

8 teaspoons (40 ml) apple cider vinegar, divided

YIELD: 2 CUPS (490 G)

In the bowl of a food processor, combine the onion and garlic. Process until finely minced, scraping down the sides of the bowl as needed. Add the cucumber, sea salt, celery seed, and mustard seed, and pulse until the desired relish texture is reached (about 10 quick pulses), scraping down as needed.

Pour the mixture into a fine-mesh strainer over a bowl. Set aside for 30 minutes to drain. After resting, discard the liquid and scoop the mixture into the now empty bowl. In a measuring cup, whisk together the honey and sauerkraut juice. Pour over the cucumber mixture and toss with a spatula to combine.

Scoop the mixture evenly into two 1-cup (235 ml) Mason jars, leaving ¾ inch (2 cm) of empty space at the top. Scoop the pulp of the relish into the jar first, then pour the juice over the top. Using the back of a spoon, push the relish down, so that the juice rises above it. Wipe down the sides and screw on the jar lid. Place in a shady spot at room temperature for 3 days, then refrigerate.

When ready to consume, fully stir 4 teaspoons (20 ml) of apple cider vinegar into each jar to arrest further fermentation.

Many ketchup recipes either require carmelizing onions before blending in the blender, which seems awfully laborious, or omitting onion altogether. By using "onion juice," which is simply the by-product of a little grated onion, the onion flavor can be included with minimal hassle.

Zesty Fermented Ketchup

2 cups (520 g) tomato paste

¼ cup (60 ml) traditional sauerkraut juice (fermented)

3 tablespoons (45 ml) sweet onion juice

2 tablespoons (40 g) raw honey

1 teaspoon sea salt

1 teaspoon garlic paste (see Note, page 69)

½ teaspoon powdered mustard

½ teaspoon allspice

¼ teaspoon cayenne, optional

2 tablespoons (30 ml) apple cider vinegar

YIELD: 3 CUPS (720 G)

In a medium-size bowl, combine all the ingredients except the vinegar. Since all tomato paste brands are different, add water, if necessary, to achieve the desired thickness. Whisk well and scoop into a 1-quart (1 L) Mason jar. Allow a ¾-inch (2 cm) empty space at the top of the jar. Seal and store at room temperature for 3 days.

After fermentation, fully stir the vinegar into the jar and refrigerate. Because vinegar slows the fermentation process, it is added after the 3-day ferment.

RECIPE NOTES

• Traditional sauerkraut juice is a nutrient-rich aid to the fermentation process. To gather the juice, simply strain a bit of sauerkraut through a small-size mesh strainer into a bowl. If homemade sauerkraut is not on hand, we suggest some store-bought varieties that will work (see Resources, page 216).

• To make onion juice, set a box grater in the center of a flat-bottomed bowl. Grate the onion over the largest holes. Scoop the resulting pulp into a small-size, fine-mesh strainer set over a measuring cup and press down on the pulp to extract the juice.

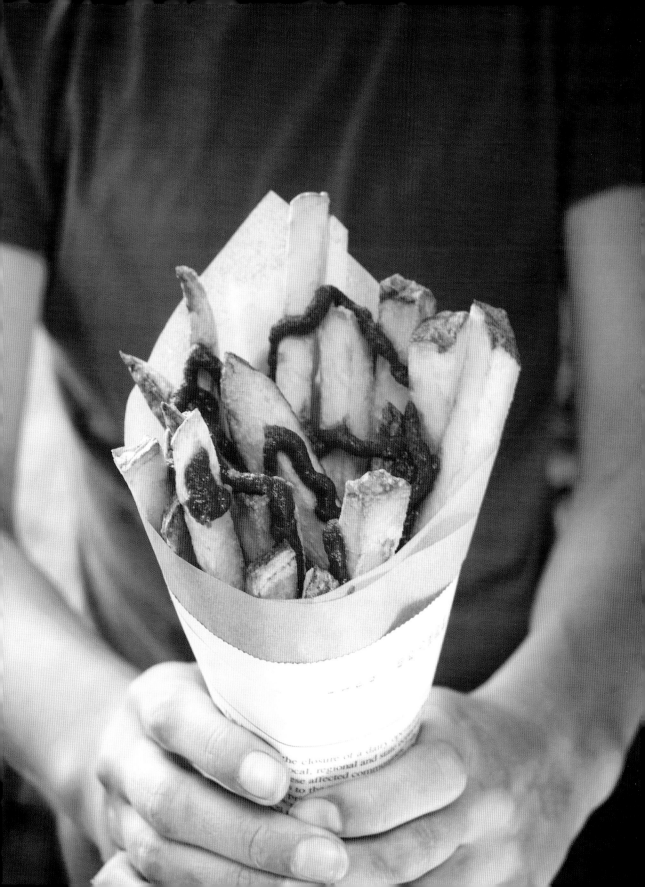

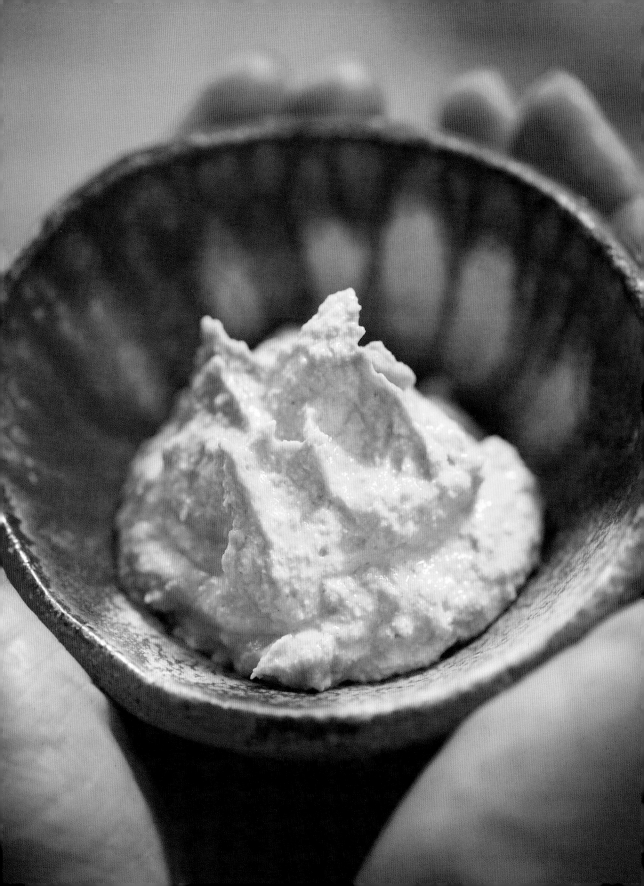

Imagine a juicy grass-fed hot dog, straight off the grill. Strong, proud, and familiar, this mustard is fermented to enhance the digestion of that dog! Traditional green cabbage sauerkraut juice, unlike the juice from the red kraut recipe (page 180), is a necessary ingredient (the red juice would turn the mustard a funky color). If homemade sauerkraut is not on hand, there are store-bought varieties that can substitute (see Resources, page 216).

Ballpark Yellow Mustard

1¼ cups (295 ml) water

1 cup (145 g) ground yellow mustard seed

2 tablespoons (30 ml) green cabbage sauerkraut juice

1 tablespoon (15 ml) lemon juice

1 tablespoon (20 g) raw honey

2 teaspoons ground turmeric

1 teaspoon sea salt

½ teaspoon crushed garlic

8 teaspoons (40 ml) apple cider vinegar

In a high-speed blender, combine the water, mustard, sauerkraut juice, lemon juice, honey, turmeric, sea salt, and garlic. Blend on high speed until smooth, about 30 to 40 seconds.

Scoop the mustard into a 1-pint (470 ml) Mason jar with a lid, leaving at least ¾ inches (2 cm) of empty space at the top of the jar. Seal and store at room temperature for 3 days.

After fermentation, fully stir the vinegar into the jar and refrigerate. Because vinegar slows the fermentation process, it is added after the 3-day ferment.

YIELD: 1 PINT (350 G)

If you're ready to take on only one homemade condiment, make it mayonnaise! I know of only one commercial variety that's reputable, and it's only available by mail order (page 217). Store-bought varieties are made with refined oils and thickening agents, but even more important, why aren't their mayonnaises yellow? It's made from egg yolks, for goodness' sake.

Simply Mayonnaise

2 egg yolks, at room temperature

2 tablespoons (30 ml) fresh lemon
  juice

½ teaspoon Dijon mustard

⅛ teaspoon sea salt

¾ cup (180 ml) extra-virgin olive oil

⅛ teaspoon freshly cracked pepper

¼ teaspoon celery seed

1 tablespoon (15 ml) whey
  (page 40), optional

In the bowl of a food processor, combine the egg yolks, lemon juice, Dijon, and sea salt. Process until combined, about 30 seconds. While the motor is running, stream the olive oil through the food processor shoot drop by drop. It is important that the oil be added very slowly, allowing each addition to fully combine and emulsify before adding the next. Once ½ cup (120 ml) of the oil has been added, oil may be added at a slightly increased speed.

Once all the oil has been incorporated, stir in the pepper celery seed, and whey, if using. If whey has been added, store in a sealed Mason jar for 7 hours at room temperature before transferring to the refrigerator. Lacto-fermentation will add probiotic benefits and extend shelf life. If not adding whey, refrigerate immediately.

Chill thoroughly before use; mayonnaise will thicken as it chills. The whey-less version may be stored in the refrigerator for at least 2 weeks; the lacto-fermented version will keep for 2 months or more in the fridge.

YIELD: ¾ CUP (170 G)

RECIPE NOTES

• Shop for an extra-virgin olive oil that is light and buttery. If the flavor is too strong, unrefined sunflower oil can be a suitable substitute.

• The key to this recipe is to very slowly drizzle in the olive oil. To make this step easy, notice the food processor chute insert has a small hole in the bottom. Simply fill with oil and watch it drip slowly.

• Sweet Mayonnaise Variation: Add 1 tablespoon (15 g) Sweet Pickle Relish (page 173) and 2 tablespoons (40 g) raw honey and whisk to combine.

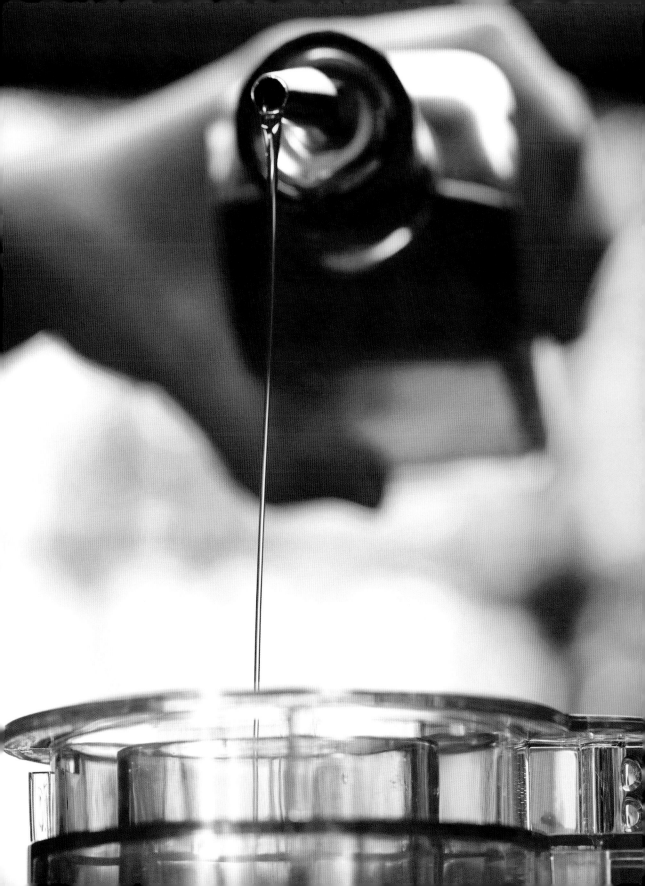

Ultimately, fermented foods, such as kraut (a.k.a. sauerkraut), should be eaten with every meal in order to properly assist digestion. Although this recipe may be eaten after a week of room-temperature fermentation, the kraut is best when allowed to continue to slowly ferment in the refrigerator for one or two additional months. The longer it ferments, the more probiotics infuse and break down this living food!

Red Cabbage Kraut with Fresh Dill

1 medium head red cabbage
¼ cup (60 ml) fresh lemon juice
1 tablespoon (4 g) chopped fresh dill and/or 1 teaspoon minced garlic
1 teaspoon sea salt
½ cup (120 ml) water

YIELD: 1 QUART (568 G)

Pull off and set aside one outer leaf of the red cabbage. Using a knife, roughly chop the cabbage into approximately 1-inch (2.5 cm) pieces, resulting in 6 cups (420 g) loosely packed chopped cabbage, a perfect amount to fit in a 1-quart (1 L) Mason jar. If the cabbage yields too much, simply store the excess for another use.

Divide the cabbage into 2 batches and, in the bowl of a food processer fitted with the traditional blade attachment, finely chop, scraping down the sides as necessary. Once processed, combine both batches in a large-size wooden or stainless steel bowl. Add the lemon juice, dill (and/or garlic), and sea salt. Toss well with a spatula to combine.

Using your fists, the blunt top of a meat mallet, or a wooden pounder, pound the cabbage mixture for about 10 minutes, until a generous amount of juice is released. Pour the water over the top of the cabbage and toss well with a spatula to combine.

Pack the mixture into a 1-quart (1 L) Mason jar that has been cleaned thoroughly with hot, soapy water. A wide-mouth canning funnel aids this process. Press the cabbage down into the jar firmly with your fist, a spoon, or a pounder until the juices rise above the cabbage. Check to make sure the top of the cabbage is at least 1½ inches (3.8 cm) below the top of the jar. If not, remove some. Clean the rim of the jar with a clean cloth or paper towel.

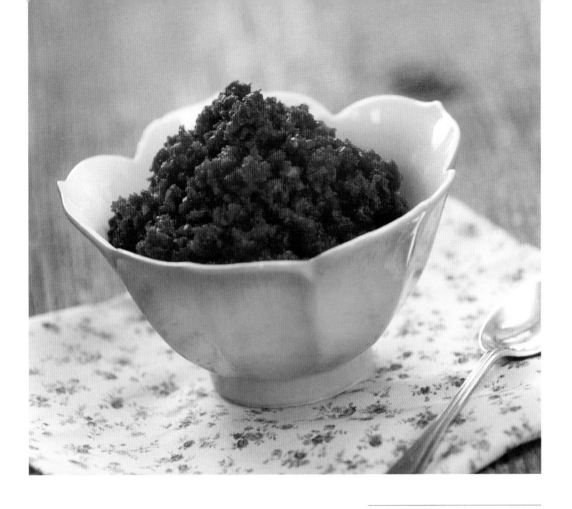

Rinse the reserved cabbage leaf, and with kitchen shears, cut from the leaf a circle slightly larger than the circumference of the jar. Push the circle down into the jar, covering the shredded cabbage. Gently press down, allowing a bit of juice to flow over the top of the cabbage leaf. The leaf edges will rest against the edges of the jar and seal in the cabbage.

Cover and place in a shaded space at room temperature for 1 week. After 1 week, transfer to the refrigerator for 1 to 2 (optional) months.

The kraut may be eaten after 1 week of fermentation. Remove the lid and discard the cabbage leaf. If any mold sits on the top of the cabbage, scoop off and discard. A thin layer of mold does not mean the batch has spoiled. Start with a teaspoon of kraut with each meal, working up to a tablespoon or more to suit your body.

RECIPE NOTE

Quality sea salt (page 216) still contains the micronutrients of the sea, which are refined away from conventional table salt. Sea salt also encourages the growth of beneficial bacteria needed for proper fermentation and controls the growth of the bad microorganisms. Refined table salt contains additives that inhibit this natural fermentation process. Sea salt is best!

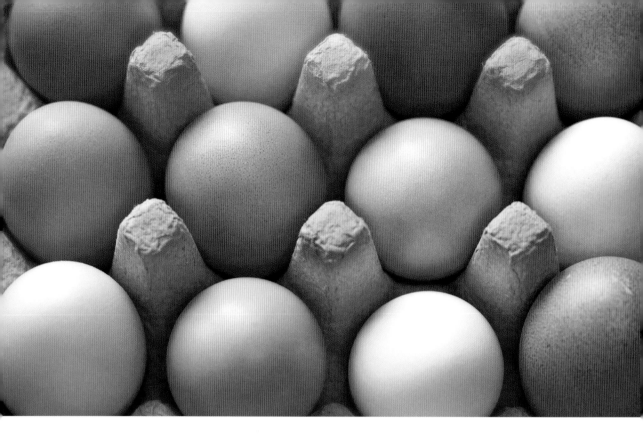

CHAPTER 12

BREAD & BREAKFAST

BUTTER IS BACK! And, we'd like to give you something good on which to spread it. My mom and I are as much alike as we are different, but there's one constant: a true love of real, grass-fed butter spread thickly across a warm slice of authentic sourdough bread.

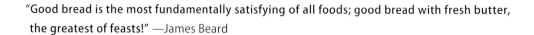

"Good bread is the most fundamentally satisfying of all foods; good bread with fresh butter, the greatest of feasts!" —James Beard

back to butter

Every cook needs a basic muffin recipe that can be whipped up in a pinch or used as a jumping-off point for any number of variations. Below is our offering to your traditional kitchen. Go wild!

Basic Sprouted Grain Muffins

½ cup (112 g) butter

½ cup (160 g) raw honey

3 cups (360 g) fresh-milled, sprouted whole wheat pastry flour (page 55)

1 teaspoon sea salt

2 teaspoons baking soda

2 teaspoons baking powder

1 egg, beaten

1 cup (235 ml) buttermilk (page 44)

YIELD: 18 MUFFINS

Preheat the oven to 400°F (200°C, or gas mark 6). Line 18 standard muffin cups with paper liners.

Combine the butter and honey in a small-size saucepan over medium heat, heating until just melted. Stir and set aside to cool.

In a large-size bowl, combine the flour, sea salt, baking soda, and baking powder, whisking briefly. In a separate bowl, add the egg to the buttermilk and whisk to combine. Add the honey mixture and buttermilk mixture to the dry ingredients, whisking until just blended.

Using a large-size cookie scoop, fill each muffin cup three-fourths full. Bake for 13 minutes, or until a toothpick inserted into the center of a muffin comes out clean.

RECIPE NOTES

• Try adding your favorite fruit to this recipe, such as blueberries or chopped peaches or pears! We recommend adding a total of 1 cup (150 g) to the final batter. Or, add a warm spike of flavor with 1 teaspoon ground cinnamon or vanilla extract.

• Using a stoneware muffin pan will add 2 minutes to the baking time.

Walnuts, when added to the batter of a muffin, often go a bit soft, which isn't bad (think walnuts in banana bread), but we like to keep some bite, so we put them on top instead, giving you the perfect mouthful of soft muffin and crunchy top. What's not to love?!

Banana-Date Sprouted Muffins

½ cup (112 g) butter

½ cup (160 g) raw honey

3 cups (360 g) fresh-milled, sprouted whole wheat pastry flour (page 55)

1 teaspoon sea salt

2 teaspoons (9 g) baking soda

2 teaspoons (9 g) baking powder

¾ cup (135 g) well packed pitted and roughly chopped Medjool dates

1 egg, beaten

1 teaspoon vanilla extract

1 cup (235 ml) buttermilk (page 44)

¾ cup (170 g) mashed ripe banana (about 2)

1 cup (150 g) finely chopped crunchy walnuts (page 49)

YIELD: 2 DOZEN MUFFINS

Preheat the oven to 400°F (200°C, or gas mark 6). Line 2 standard muffin tins with paper liners.

Melt the butter and honey in a small-size saucepan over medium heat. Stir and set aside to cool.

Measure the flour into a large-size mixing bowl, then remove 1 tablespoon (8 g) to be combined with the dates in the next step. Add the sea salt, baking soda, and baking powder to the large-size bowl and whisk briefly to combine. Set aside.

Place the chopped dates in a small-size bowl and sprinkle with the reserved flour. Using your fingers, separate and cover dates with flour. Set aside.

Add the egg and vanilla to the buttermilk, whisking to combine. Add the honey mixture, buttermilk mixture, and mashed banana to the dry ingredients, whisking until just blended. With a spatula, fold in the dates.

Using a large-size cookie scoop, fill each muffin cup three-fourths full. Sprinkle the top of each muffin with a scant spoonful of walnuts. Bake for 13 to 15 minutes, or until a toothpick inserted into the center of a muffin comes out clean.

RECIPE NOTE

Before measuring the honey, grease the inside of the measuring cup with a bit of butter or olive oil; this will allow the honey to pour more easily from the cup without sticking.

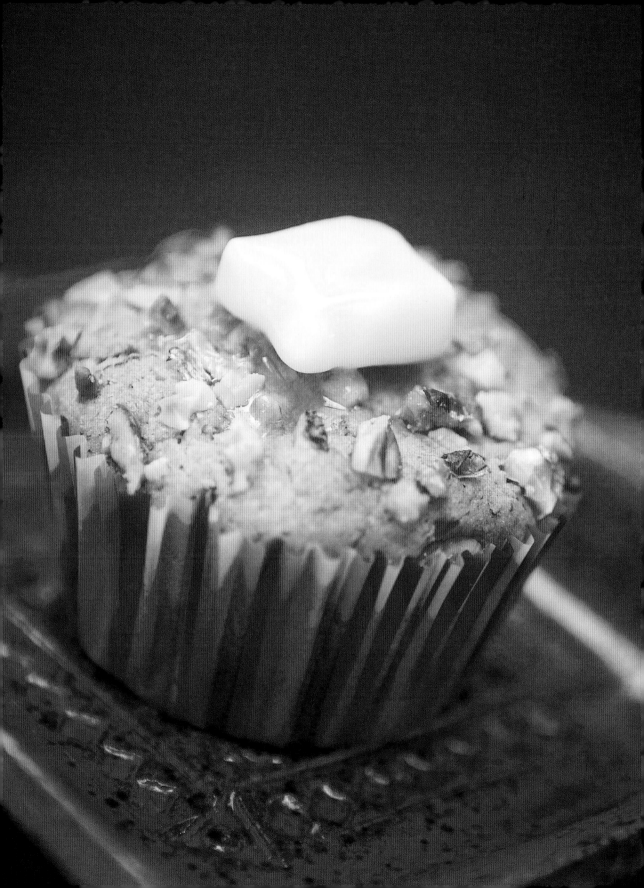

Because the eggs are without refrigeration during the fermentation process, some people avoid using them as an ingredient in sourdough bread. I enjoy the texture and flavor that eggs lend to bread too much to leave them out, and I also use pastured eggs from our farm, which causes me not to fear. I encourage you to seek out local, pastured eggs in order to try this recipe with confidence. Note that there is a minimum of 12 hours of advance prep time.

Rustic Sourdough Bread

½ cup (120 ml) rye starter (page 57), recently fed and bubbly

1 cup (120 g) fresh-milled rye flour (unsprouted)

1⅓ cups (320 ml) water, divided

⅓ cup (75 g) butter, softened

¼ cup (80 g) raw honey

2 eggs, beaten

2 teaspoons sea salt

4 cups (480 g) fresh-milled, sprouted, whole wheat bread flour (page 55), plus more for dusting and kneading

YIELD: ONE (10-INCH, OR 25 CM) ROUND LOAF

The night before breadmaking, prepare the pre-ferment by combining the starter, rye flour, and ⅔ cup (160 ml) of the water in the bowl of a standing mixer. Stir and cover with plastic wrap. Set aside in a warm spot for 12 hours; an oven with the light on and the door cracked works well.

The following morning, combine the pre-ferment, the remaining ⅔ cup (160 ml) water, butter, honey, eggs, and sea salt. Mix using the dough hook on the STIR setting to combine. Add the bread flour and knead in the mixer, continuing to use the STIR setting for 12 minutes. The dough will become smoother and slightly dense, but will still be too loose and sticky to shape into a ball. Remove the bowl from the mixer and cover with a tea towel. Set aside in a warm, draft-free place for 4 hours, or until doubled in size.

While the dough is rising, prepare for the next step. If you have a banneton (a linen-lined basket specifically for breadmaking), pull that out, or have ready a large-size colander or bowl and line it with a thin flour sack tea towel. Using sprouted whole wheat flour, liberally dust either the linen of the banneton or the flour sack tea towel with flour. Be generous with your flouring; you do not want the bread to stick to the towel during its second rise. Set aside.

Once the dough has doubled, sprinkle additional sprouted bread flour onto a cutting board and coat your clean hands with flour. Plop the dough onto the floured surface. Dust with

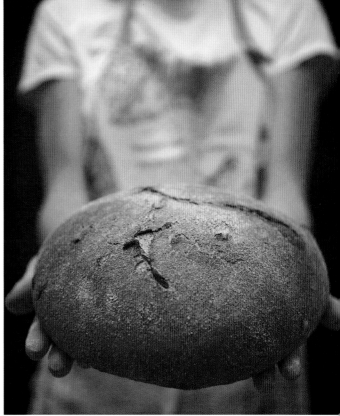

a little more flour and begin to gently knead the dough by hand. You will knead for no more than a minute. Add only enough flour to shape the dough into a ball and no more! It is very important to limit the amount of flour used in this step. As soon as the dough can be formed into a ball without completely sticking to your hands (it will still be lightly tacky), place the dough, pretty side down, into the prepared towel-lined bowl or banneton. Cover with another tea towel and set aside to rise for 2 hours. Sourdough bread does not rise quite as high during the second rise as conventional yeast bread does, but do not be alarmed; it will rise further in the oven.

A half hour before the dough is finished rising, Have ready a 7-quart (6.3 L) stainless steel, cast-iron, or enameled pot with a tight-fitting lid—whatever you use, be sure it's oven-safe up to at least 450°F (230°C, or gas mark 8). Adjust the racks of the oven so that the pot will sit exactly in the center when baking. Place the pot, with its lid, into the oven as it is preheating.

Gently flip the dough into the hot pot, being careful not to puncture or deflate the bread. Cover with the lid and bake for 15 minutes, then lower the heat to 400ºF (200ºC, or gas mark 6) and bake for an additional 30 minutes, until the bread has a browned, sturdy crust with a crispy bottom.

Remove the pot from the oven, uncover, and let rest for 5 minutes. Carefully remove the bread from the pan and cool on wire rack before slicing.

RECIPE NOTE

Try a caramelized onion loaf! While the bread is in its first rise, heat a large-size cast-iron skillet over medium heat. Add 1 tablespoon (14 g) butter and 2 cups (320 g) sliced onion. When the butter melts, stir. Reduce the heat to low and continue to stir every 5 minutes for the next 30 minutes, until golden brown and caramelized. Remove from the heat and scoop into a bowl. Set aside until the bread is ready.

After the first rise, plop the dough onto a floured board, and kneed briefly, as described in the instructions. Spread out the dough into an 8-inch (20 cm) round circle and spread the caramelized onions evenly over the surface, then fold over and knead for 1 minute, as called for. Continue with the recipe per usual.

bread & breakfast

Sourcing or making authentic sourdough bread, whose rise originates from a natural sourdough starter, enables the cook to produce high-quality bread crumbs. Don't expect these crumbs to be the granular texture of the store-bought variety, however, which typically contain loads of additives. Instead, they will be bready, not sandy—more like small, delicious snowflakes.

Sourdough Bread Crumbs

10 cups (500 g) lightly packed cubed Rustic Sourdough Bread (with crust) (page 186)
1 teaspoon sea salt, divided
½ teaspoon freshly cracked black pepper, divided

YIELD: 6 CUPS (300 G)

RECIPE NOTE

The fluffy texture of these bread crumbs shine in our Fresh Herb–Crusted Sea Bass (page 118) and Mom's Meatloaf (page 146). If purchasing a loaf of sourdough bread to make these crumbs, make sure yeast is not an ingredient, because it signals the use of *commercial yeast*, instead of authentic *sourdough starter*. The basic ingredients for a simple sourdough bread are flour, water, and sea salt; any additional ingredients should be real food ingredients used to create flavor or texture, such as honey, eggs, olives, or nuts.

Preheat the oven to 300ºF (150ºC, or gas mark 2). Spread the cubed bread on a cookie sheet. Bake for 10 minutes without turning. Remove, and set aside to cool for 10 minutes. The bread cubes will be soft, resulting in a "stale" texture that hardens a bit as it cools, but maintains a slight give when squeezed.

In a food processor, combine half the toasted and cooled bread, ½ teaspoon of the sea salt, and ¼ teaspoon of the pepper. Process for 1 minute, until the crumbs are about the size of peas or smaller (lack of uniformity in size is fine); do not process all the way to a sandy texture. The crumbs will maintain a bread-like texture, sticking together when squeezed. If any awkward large chunks remain, pulse to the desired texture. Pour into a large-size bowl and repeat with the second batch of toasted bread and the remaining ½ teaspoon sea salt and ¼ teaspoon pepper. Add to the first batch and toss to combine.

Store in a sealed container until use. For long-term storage, store in the freezer.

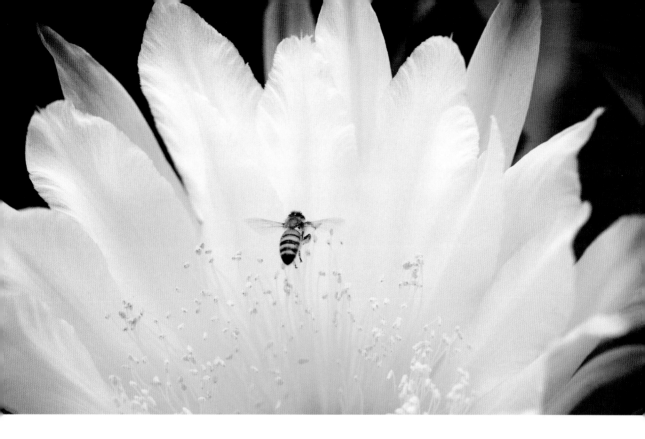

CHAPTER 13

SAVE ROOM FOR DESSERT!

NOT ONLY DO REFINED SUGARS AND FLOURS OFFER NOTHING NUTRITIONALLY, but let's be honest—they're also boring! Diversity and depth of flavor are pushed aside, leaving behind—white. Reminds me of Apricot Lane Farms, before our land was transfomred. The soil was sandy and barren, kind of like refined soil. The former farmer limited all life except for the desired crop—no weeds, no bugs, no animals. Conversely, our biodynamic method enlists diversity and life to support health and vitality! These days the farm feels full and complex, just like a raw clover honey or a mineral-rich maple syrup.

A QUICK NOTE ON FLOUR: All recipes calling for flour in this chapter have been created using fresh-milled flour (often sprouted), which creates a very light, airy texture. Dense, store-bought flour will not produce the same result.

The casual, homey, and economical nature of this recipe falls perfectly in line with our historical food genes, and gives one last breath of life to stale bread. My dad loves this dish. He scoops it into a bowl and drowns it with raw milk. Highly recommended!

Sourdough Bread Pudding with Raisins

2 eggs
½ cup (100 g) maple sugar (page 65)
2 cups (470 ml) milk
¼ teaspoon sea salt
1½ teaspoons vanilla extract
1 teaspoon cinnamon
2 cups (100 g) 1-inch (2.5 cm) cubed day-old Rustic Sourdough Bread (page 186)
¾ cup (110 g) raisins

YIELD: 6 SERVINGS

Preheat the oven to 350ºF (180ºC, or gas mark 4). Have ready an 8 x 8-inch (20 x 20 cm) glass baking dish and a 9 x 13-inch (23 x 33 cm) glass baking dish (no need to grease).

In a large-size bowl, add the eggs and whisk for 30 seconds. Add the maple sugar and whisk for about 30 seconds to begin dissolving the crystals. Add the milk, sea salt, vanilla, and cinnamon and stir until the maple sugar is fully dissolved. Lastly, fold in the bread cubes and raisins with the spatula.

Pour the mixture into the ungreased 8 x 8-inch (20 x 20 cm) dish. Set that dish inside the 9 x 13-inch (23 x 33 cm) dish. Fill the 9 x 13-inch (23 x 33 cm) dish with 1 inch (2.5 cm) of hot tap water, taking care not to spill water into the bread pudding. This creates a water bath, which will prevent the custard portion of the bread pudding from burning. Place the whole contraption into the oven and bake for 1 hour. When done, the milk custard on the bottom will be congealed and tips of the bread poking through will be lightly browned.

Remove the pudding from the oven and from its water bath and allow it to cool slightly. Serve hot or cold.

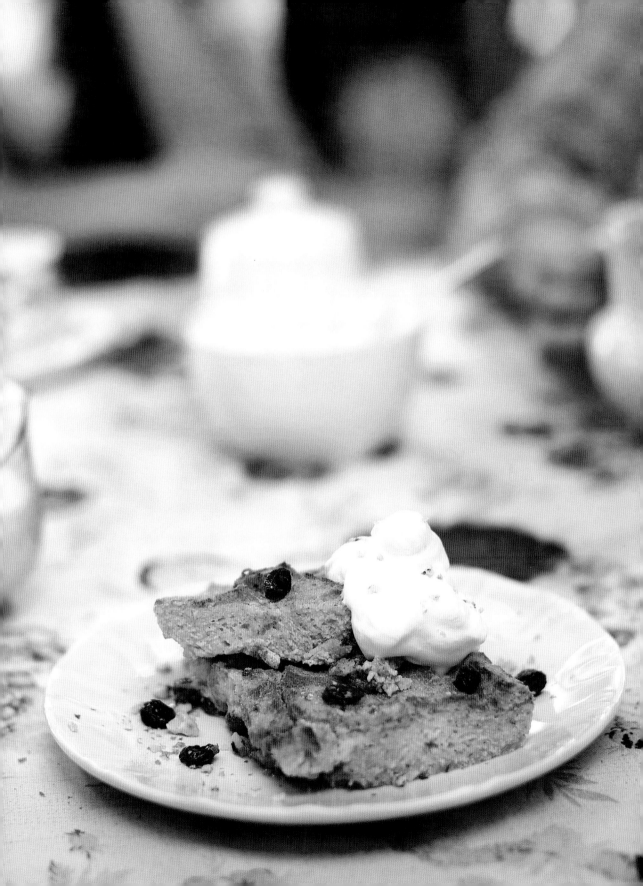

Before becoming a farmer myself, I was a private chef, and I worked for a family on their farm in Santa Barbara, California. Unknowingly planting the seeds of my future, I vividly remember setting out to pick peaches to make this very cobbler. Peaches are perfection in this recipe, but my mom has also successfully used farm-fresh blackberries. We encourage experimentation!

Crispy Peach Cobbler

6 tablespoons (84 g) butter

2 cups (340 g) peeled and sliced peaches

⅔ cup (105 g) honey granules (page 64)

1 teaspoon cinnamon

1 teaspoon almond extract

1¼ cups (150 g) fresh-milled, sprouted whole wheat pastry flour (page 55)

2 teaspoons (9 g) baking powder

⅛ teaspoon sea salt

¾ cup (180 ml) milk

YIELD: 6 SERVINGS

RECIPE NOTE

Fresh or frozen peaches both work well here. If using frozen, thaw before using. Some juice from the thawed (or fresh) peaches is necessary to begin dissolving the honey granules, but you only need about 2 tablespoons (30 ml) to get the job done, so strain (or drink) the rest before beginning. Too much juice has a tendency to cause the dough to become gooey.

Preheat the oven to 350ºF (180ºC, or gas mark 4). Place the butter in a 7 x 11-inch (17.8 x 28 cm) glass or ceramic baking dish and put the dish into the oven while it preheats, for about 10 minutes, allowing the butter to melt, but not brown.

Meanwhile, in a medium-size bowl, combine the sliced peaches, honey granules, cinnamon, and almond extract. Stir to combine and set aside.

In a second medium-size bowl, combine the flour, baking powder, and sea salt. Whisk to combine.

When the butter is melted, remove the pan from the oven and set aside. The next step will cause the dough to rise quickly, so be sure to finish all of the above tasks first and work quickly.

Add the milk to the flour mixture and whisk together quickly. Scoop over the melted butter in the pan as evenly as possible. There is no need to spread the batter because it will spread as it bakes. Carefully spoon the sweetened fruit, along with 2 tablespoons (30 ml) of the juice in the bowl, evenly over the flour mixture.

Bake for 40 minutes, until the dough is a light golden brown. Serve warm with fresh whipped cream or a scoop of ice cream.

This recipe uses a piping bag, which is the tool bakers use to decorate cakes. In my opinion, the easiest way to fill one is to set the bag tip-side down in a tall glass and fold the ends of the bag over the sides of the glass. Scoop the mixture into the bag, then take out and twist the bag just above the top of its contents to push the mixture down into the tip. In the heat of the summer months, you may want to stick these chips in the fridge to prevent melting. But overall, they are shelf-stable. Note that there is 6 hours of advance prep time.

Soy-Free Carob Chips

1½ cups (225 g) raw cashews

2⅛ teaspoons (12.75 g) sea salt, divided

½ cup (120 ml) coconut milk

2 tablespoons (16 g) bovine gelatin

¼ cup (80 g) raw honey

2 teaspoons (10 ml) vanilla extract

½ cup (112 g) solid coconut oil

1 cup (120 g) roasted carob powder

YIELD: 4 CUPS (700 G)

RECIPE NOTES

• Roasted carob powder can be found at most health food stores.

• For quality gelatin, see Resources (page 216) for purchasing suggestions.

In a medium-size bowl, combine the cashews, 2 teaspoons (12 g) of the sea salt, and enough water to cover by 2 inches (5 cm). Set aside for 6 hours. After soaking, pour the cashews into a mesh colander and rinse and drain thoroughly.

Whisk the coconut milk and gelatin together in a small-size bowl, combining thoroughly. Set aside.

In the bowl of a food processor, combine the soaked cashews, honey, vanilla, and remaining ⅛ teaspoon sea salt. Process the mixture for 2 minutes, scraping down the sides with a spatula as necessary. Add the coconut oil and coconut milk/gelatin mixture and process for an additional 2 minutes. Add the carob powder and process for an additional 1 minute, or until the mixture is smooth and creamy. Grains of cashews will still be apparent, but they should be very small, like grains of sand. Allow the mixture to stand for 5 minutes.

Have ready 2 nonstick dehydrator sheets with racks while the mixture rests. After 5 minutes, scoop the mixture into a piping bag fitted with a number 5 tip, if you have it, or a freezer bag with a small tip cut off one corner. Pipe rows of little chocolate chips onto the sheets. This is a very tedious process. Turn on some good music and settle in!

Dehydrate chips at 135ºF (57ºC) for 12 hours. Cool and store in a sealed container at room temperature.

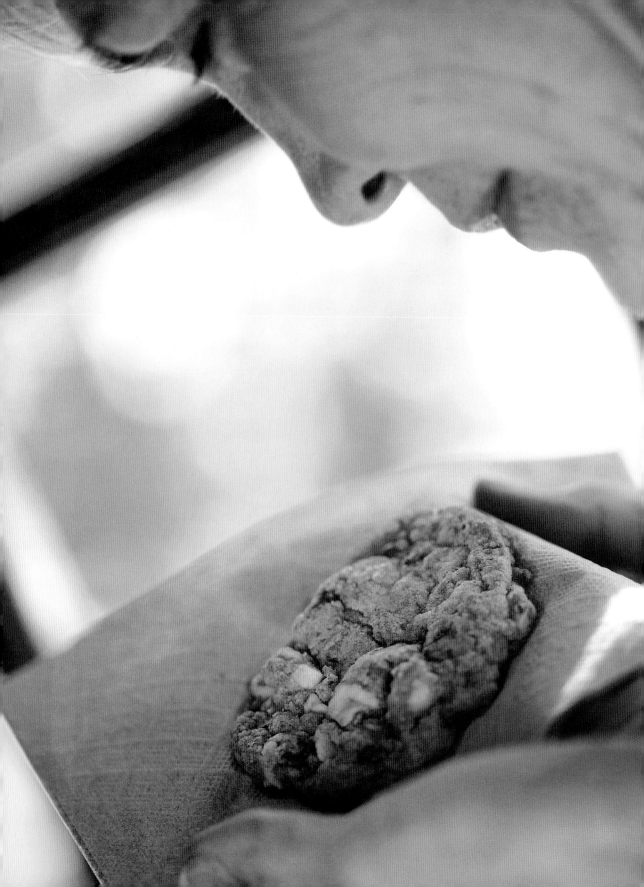

We've found that switching from chocolate chips to carob chips eliminates the highs and lows created by the caffeine in chocolate, especially for kids. Store-bought carob chips are delicious, but they contain soy. If you are soy-sensitive like me, try making our soy-free version at home. Our family stores these cookies in the freezer. It enhances their crunch and extends the life of this preservative-free treat.

Chips Off the Old Block

1 cup (225 g) butter, softened

1 cup (160 g) honey granules (page 64)

1 cup (200 g) Sucanat (page 64)

2 eggs

1 teaspoon vanilla extract

1½ cups (180 g) fresh-milled, sprouted whole wheat pastry flour (page 55)

1½ cups (180 g) fresh-milled, sprouted whole wheat bread flour (page 55)

1 teaspoon baking soda

1 teaspoon baking powder

½ teaspoon sea salt

1 cup (150 g) roughly chopped crunchy walnuts or pecans (page 49), optional

2 cups (350 g) Soy-Free Carob Chips (page 193)

YIELD: 3 DOZEN COOKIES

Preheat the oven to 350°F (180ºC, or gas mark 4). Line 3 cookie sheets with parchment paper.

In the bowl of an electric mixer, gradually cream together the butter, honey granules, and Sucanat to make a grainy paste. Add the eggs and vanilla and beat well.

In a medium-size bowl, combine the flours, baking soda, baking powder, and sea salt. Whisk briefly to combine. Gradually add to the creamed ingredients, about 1 cup (120 g) at a time, until combined. Add the nuts and carob chips. Mix again to combine.

Using a 1½-inch (3.8 cm) cookie scoop or two spoons, form the dough into balls and place 2 inches (5 cm) apart on the prepared cookie sheets, 12 to a sheet. (Tip: Dipping the scoop into a cup of ice water helps facilitate the release of the dough.)

Bake one tray at time for 10 to 12 minutes each. Each cookie will spread to about 2½ inches (6.4 cm) and be a nice deep brown once baked.

Cool on the pan for 3 to 4 minutes before transferring to a cooling rack.

As the name suggests, Chester Cookies are a staple in my house. These "cookies" are so healthy they can literally be eaten for breakfast. A traditional soaking technique is introduced below, so be sure to read the instructions carefully. The oats are soaked overnight, which greatly increases their digestibility. Cool the cookies completely before storing in an airtight container. Chester Cookies are even better the second day! Note that there is a minimum of 12 hours of advance prep time.

Chester Cookies

2 cups (160 g) rolled oats

1 cup (235 ml) plain kefir (page 42)

5 tablespoons (70 g) butter, softened

2 eggs

¾ cup (195 g) almond butter (page 50)

1 teaspoon cinnamon

1 teaspoon sea salt

1 teaspoon green powdered stevia (page 65)

1½ cups (225 g) small diced green apple

½ cup (75 g) currants

½ cup (75 g) chopped crunchy walnuts (page 49)

½ cup (40 g) unsweetened coconut, optional

½ cup (88 g) Soy-Free Carob Chips (page 193), optional

YIELD: 3½ DOZEN COOKIES

The night before baking, place the oats into a clean, glass bowl. Add the kefir and stir until fully combined. Cover with a clean tea towel and set aside until morning, or 12 hours. Place the butter in a small-size bowl to soften, cover, and go to bed!

When ready to bake, preheat the oven to 350°F (180°C, or gas mark 4). Line 3 cookie sheets with parchment paper. To the kefir-oat mixture, add the eggs, softened butter, almond butter, cinnamon, sea salt, and stevia. With a hand mixer, beat until fully combined. Add the apple, currants, walnuts, coconut, and carob chips and beat again until just combined.

Using a 1½-inch (3.8 cm) cookie scoop or two spoons, drop cookies onto the prepared cookie sheets, leaving 1 inch (2.5 cm) between each (these cookies don't spread much in the oven).

Bake for 12 to 14 minutes, or until the bottoms are beautifully browned—the crunchy bottom is important. Serve warm or cooled.

RECIPE NOTE

If you can't tolerate stevia, ¼ cup (60 ml) maple sugar is a delicious substitute.

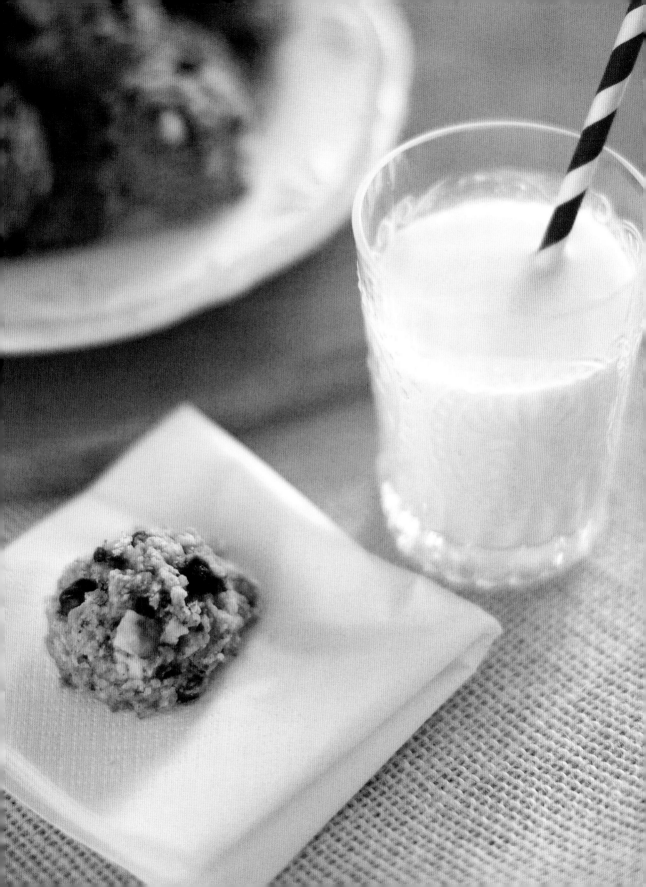

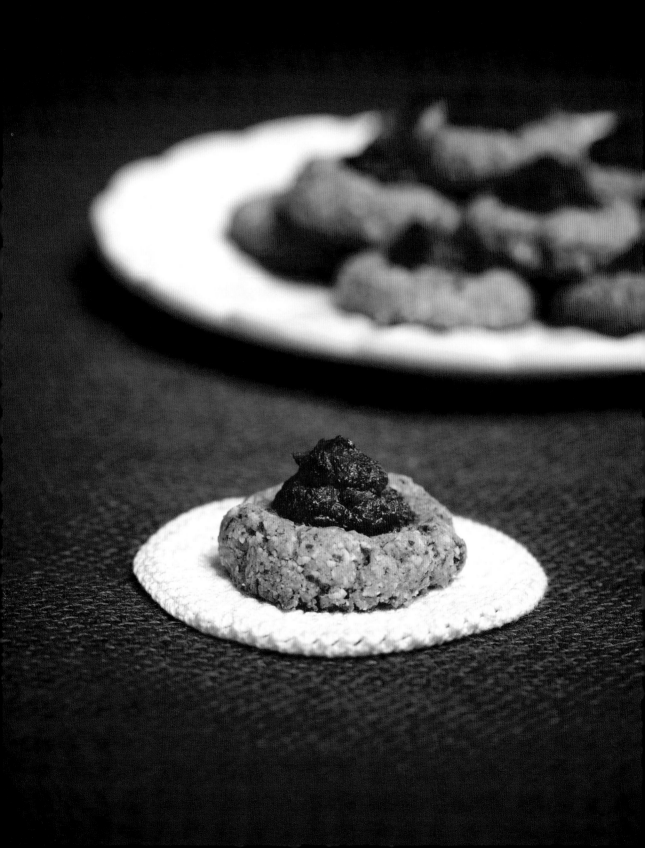

These cookies evolved from a recipe I learned in culinary school at the Natural Gourmet Institute of Culinary Arts in New York City. At every open house, the school serves their take on a classic Jam Dot Cookie. A friend of mine said she actually chose to attend the school because of those cookies! Our Sprouted Apple Butter Dots are a bit different with sprouted whole wheat flour and coarsely chopped raisins, but we're certain they still contain their own Jam Dot magic.

Sprouted Apple Butter Dots

1½ cups (225 g) crunchy almonds (page 49)

1½ cups (180 g) fresh-milled, sprouted whole wheat pastry flour (page 55)

1 teaspoon cinnamon

1 teaspoon sea salt

½ cup (120 ml) maple syrup

½ cup (112 g) coconut oil, melted

1 cup (145 g) coarsely chopped raisins

Scant ½ cup (160 g) unsweetened apple butter

YIELD: 20 COOKIES

Preheat the oven to 350ºF (180ºC, or gas mark 4) and line 2 cookie sheets with parchment paper.

In a food processor, grind the almonds into a coarse meal. Pour into a medium-size bowl and add the flour, cinnamon, and sea salt. Whisk to combine.

In a separate, small-size bowl, whisk together the maple syrup and melted coconut oil. Pour over the flour mixture and stir well to combine. Add the raisins, stirring to combine.

Form the dough into balls, slightly larger than a walnut, and place on the prepared cookie sheets, about 2 inches (5 cm) apart. Using your thumb, press an indentation into the center of each cookie. The dough may crack, and if so, simply press to repair for a more uniform look, or leave cracked for a more rustic look. Scoop 1 teaspoon apple butter into the center of each cookie.

Bake for 12 minutes, or until the bottoms are nicely browned.

RECIPE NOTE

Both blanched and regular almonds are delicious in this recipe. Blanched almonds result in a crisper cookie. You can also try pecans, which result in a richer taste and slightly moister end result.

These cookies have been a family favorite since forever, but replacing the white flour and sugar with sprouted flour and natural sweetener was risky business and no easy task! But we did it! Keep in mind, the sour cream makes them even moister the second day.

Old-Fashioned Sour Cream Drops

FOR FROSTING:

6 tablespoons (84 g) butter

2 cups (320 g) powdered honey granules (page 64)

3 tablespoons (45 ml) raw milk

1 tablespoon (15 ml) vanilla extract

FOR COOKIES:

½ cup (112 g) butter, softened

1½ cups (240 g) honey granules (page 64)

2 eggs

1 cup (225 g) sour cream

1 teaspoon vanilla extract

4 cups (480 g) fresh-milled, sprouted whole wheat pastry flour (page 55), divided

1 teaspoon baking soda

1 teaspoon baking powder

1 teaspoon sea salt

YIELD: 3½ DOZEN COOKIES

TO MAKE THE FROSTING: In a small-size saucepan over medium heat, melt the butter. Combine the honey granules, milk, and vanilla in a medium-size mixing bowl and pour the hot, melted butter over the top. Blend with an electric mixer for 3 minutes. Let the frosting rest while preparing the batter and baking the cookies, allowing the honey granules to fully dissolve. Beat again briefly before frosting the cookies.

TO MAKE THE COOKIES: Preheat the oven to 350ºF (180ºC, or gas mark 4). Line 3 cookie sheets with parchment paper.

In a large-size mixing bowl, beat the butter, honey granules, and eggs with an electric mixer on low speed to combine. Beat in the sour cream and vanilla, blending well.

Add 2 cups (240 g) of the flour and the baking soda, baking powder, and sea salt and blend thoroughly. Add the remaining 2 cups (240 g) flour and blend for about 30 seconds. Chill, covered, for at least 30 minutes.

Using a 1½-inch (3.8 cm) cookie scoop, drop the batter on ungreased cookie sheets 2 inches (5 cm) apart.

Bake for 10 minutes. Do not overbake; remove just as the edges of the cookie begin to turn brown. Cool completely before frosting. Store frosted cookies in an airtight container.

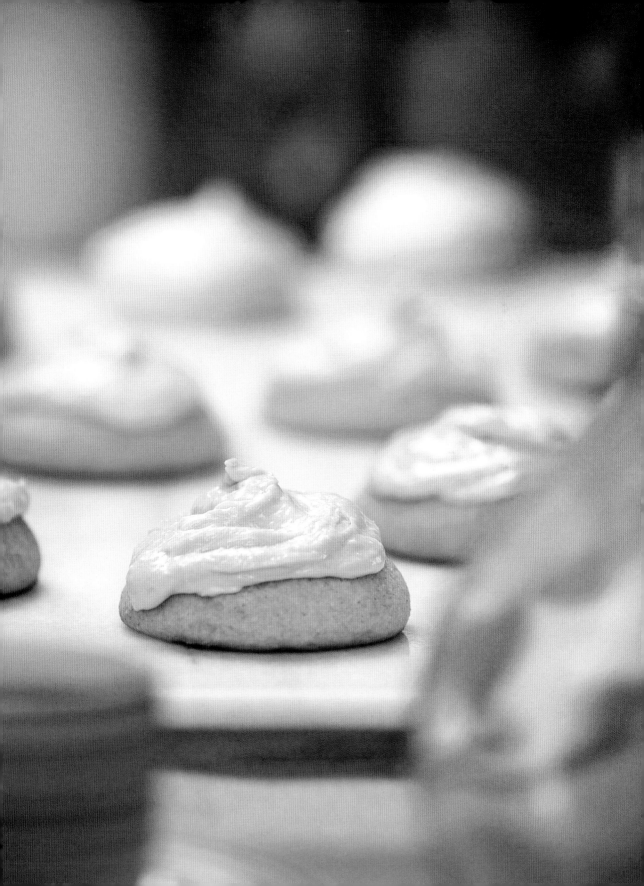

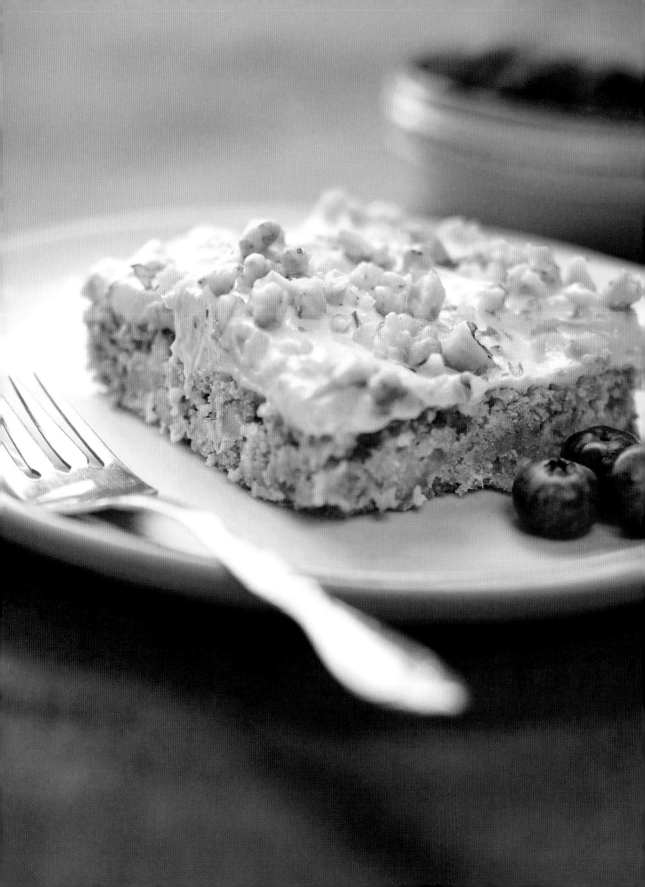

Kitchen warning! Although most recipes in this chapter call for sprouted flour, this recipe will not work with sprouted flour. Sprouting and soaking are two different techniques used to release mineral-blocking phytic acid from whole grains. If using sprouted flour, soaking is not necessary and vice versa. This cake is much better the second day. Bring to room temperature before serving. Note that there is a minimum of 12 hours of advance prep time.

Maple Walnut Cake with Cream Cheese Frosting

FOR CAKE:

1 cup (235 ml) kefir (page 42)

1½ cups (180 g) fresh-milled whole-wheat pastry flour (unsprouted) (page 55)

½ cup (40 g) rolled oats

½ cup (112 g) butter

¾ cup (150 g) maple sugar (page 65)

2 eggs

2 teaspoons (10 ml) vanilla extract

½ teaspoon sea salt

2 teaspoons (9 g) baking powder

½ cup (75 g) finely chopped crunchy walnuts (page 49)

½ cup (40 g) unsweetened shredded coconut

FOR FROSTING:

1 cup (225 g) Yogurt Cream Cheese (page 40), softened

3 tablespoons (45 ml) maple syrup

½ teaspoon vanilla extract

½ cup (75 g) finely chopped crunchy walnuts (page 49)

TO MAKE THE CAKE: The night before or 12 hours prior to baking, combine the kefir, flour, and rolled oats in a glass bowl. Stir, cover with a thin dishcloth, and set aside in a warm spot for 12 hours. Unwrap and put the butter in a medium-size bowl to soften, cover, and go to bed!

The next day, preheat the oven to 325ºF (170ºC, or gas mark 3). Butter a 7 x 11-inch (17.8 x 28 cm) glass dish.

To the bowl with the softened butter, add the maple sugar. Beat with a hand mixer on medium speed until creamy. Add the eggs, vanilla, and sea salt and beat to combine. Add the soaked flour mixture and the baking powder. Beat on medium speed for 30 seconds and on high speed for 1 minute; the mixture will be well combined, with some lumps. Add the walnuts and coconut beat to combine.

Pour into the prepared dish and bake for 35 to 40 minutes, or until a toothpick inserted into the center of the cake comes out clean. Cool completely before frosting.

TO MAKE THE FROSTING: In a medium-size bowl, combine the cream cheese, maple syrup, and vanilla. Beat well with a hand mixer on high speed. Add the walnuts and beat on low speed until just combined. Frost the cake and serve.

YIELD: 8 SERVINGS

Long ago, a very special neighbor, Mary Anne Adams, taught my mom a lot about the kitchen and even more about lasting friendships. These shortcakes were one of her offerings. The butter used to be "margarine" and the baking powder used to be "cornstarch"; however, the basic ingredient of friendship has never changed. Thank you, E-Anne.

E-Anne's Shortcakes

Inspired by Mary Anne Adams

1 cup (225 g) butter

1 teaspoon vanilla extract

½ cup (80 g) honey granules (page 64)

2¾ cups (330 g) fresh-milled, sprouted whole-wheat pastry flour (page 55)

¼ teaspoon baking powder

Fresh fruit, for serving

Freshly whipped cream or ice cream, for serving

YIELD: 8 SERVINGS

Preheat the oven to 325°F (170°C, or gas mark 3). Have ready a 7 x 11-inch (17.8 x 28 cm) glass baking dish (no need to grease).

In a small-size saucepan over medium heat, melt the butter. Remove from the heat and stir in the vanilla. Set aside.

In the bowl of a food processor, add the honey granules and process for 30 seconds. Add the flour and baking powder and pulse 2 or 3 times to combine. With the processor chute open and the motor running, pour in the melted butter mixture. Continue processing until the dough sticks together in a ball, 30 to 45 seconds. Using a rubber spatula, remove the dough from the processor and press into the baking dish.

Place on the center rack of the oven and bake for 25 minutes. After baking, remove and set aside to cool for 20 minutes.

Score the shortcake (lightly cut the surface without pressing through to the pan) into 8 equal pieces and allow to cool completely. Once cool, diagonally prick the center of each square twice with a fork. Finally, using the scored lines as guidelines, cut through the squares completely.

To serve, top each individual piece with desired topping. Plain shortcake may be stored in an airtight container at room temperature for several days.

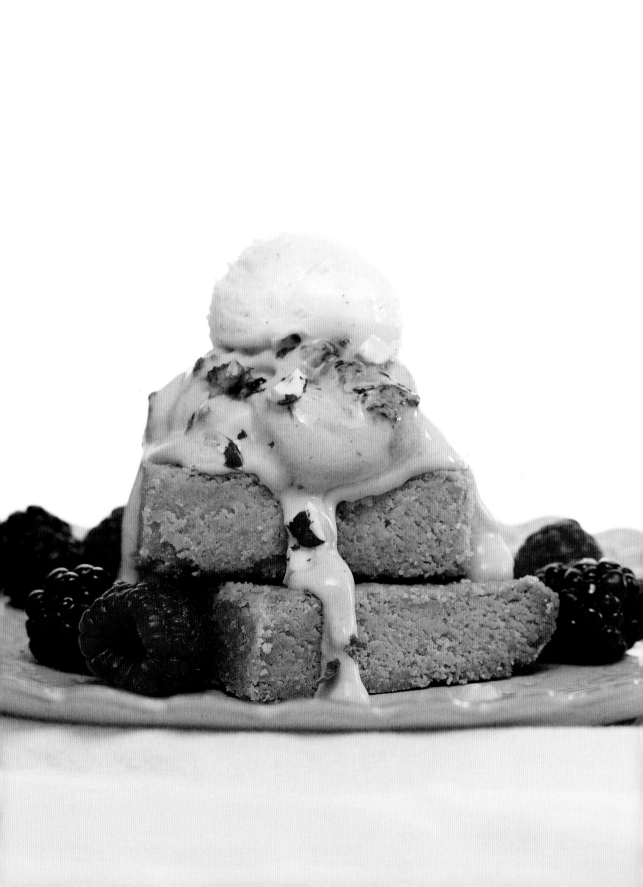

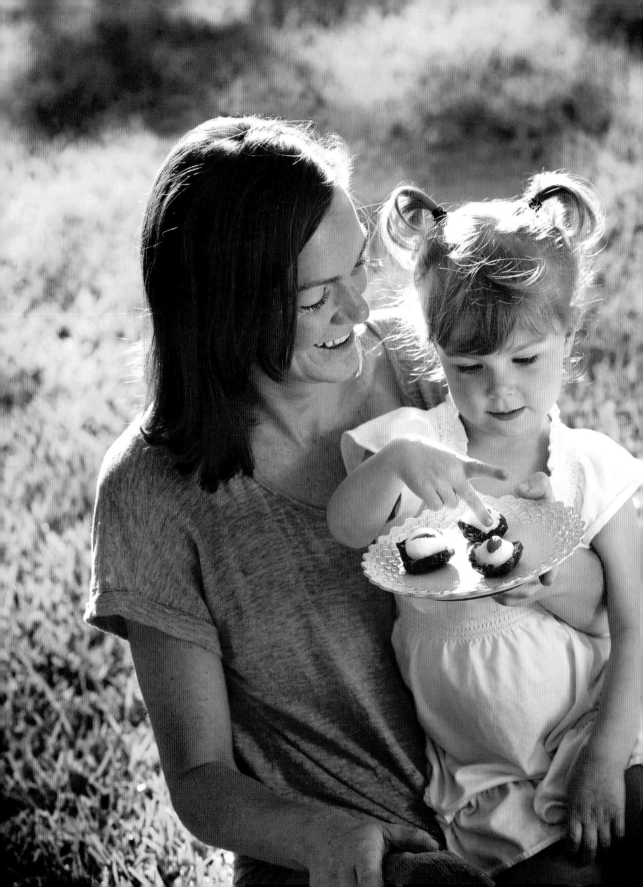

For the average day when dessert really shouldn't be on the menu, but you're dying for something sweet, here's the solution. The key ingredient is a juicy Medjool date and a bit of trust, because who would pair a date with coconut oil?! We would! It's delicious, and the coconut oil stops any craving for additional sweets in its tracks.

Almond Boy

1 large Medjool date

½ to 1 teaspoon Soy-Free Carob Chips (page 193)

1 tablespoon (14 g) coconut oil, soft but not melted

1 whole crunchy almond (page 49)

Split open and pit the date. Fill it with as many carob chips as you like. Smother the top with coconut oil. Place the almond on top and press down lightly. Enjoy!

YIELD: 1 SERVING

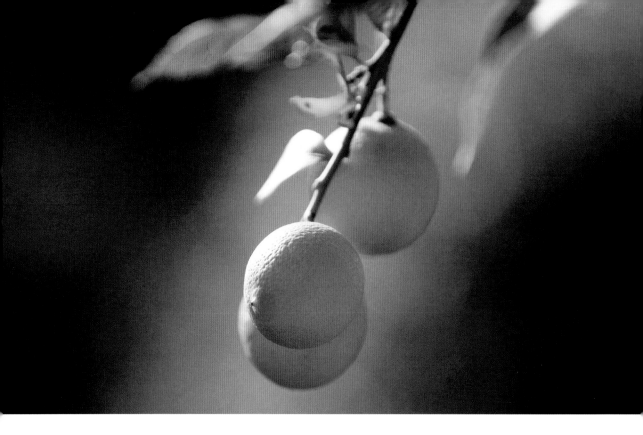

CHAPTER 14

CHEERS!

WE'D LIKE TO RAISE OUR GLASSES AND TOAST A BEVERAGE REVOLUTION. We think
we need it, folks! If we step back and take a look, our kids are currently drinking pink milk, colored and
flavored "water," and frightening amounts of juice and soda. Adults are chugging big gulp, chemically
laden "diet" drinks and coffee cocktails with more faux whipped cream and sugar-free syrup than
espresso. On top of that, we've forgotten about our fundamental need for plain old water. This chapter
offers a few delicious and health-supportive alternatives. Bottoms up!

This recipe is the one and only time you'll find evaporated cane sugar, a close cousin to refined white sugar, in our book. But the good news is that you won't be consuming it— your kombucha will! Kombucha, a traditional fermented beverage, has gained popularity in the last four years for its digestive and mood-enhancing benefits. Usually, this tea is made in single batches that take between 10 days to 3 weeks to brew, which forces the cook to clean everything out and start over each time. Below, we teach you how to maintain a continuous brew, which is decanted halfway every 7 days and refilled without ever (or very rarely) having to clean out the vessel. Note that you'll need a 2½-gallon (9.5 L) porcelain vessel with a plastic spigot and loose-leaf tea (see Resources, page 216), for this recipe.

Continuous Brew Kombucha

Inspired by Hannah Crum and Monica Ford

FOR STARTER BATCH:

8 cups (1880 ml) water

8 tablespoons (64 g) loose black (or green) tea

2 cups (400 g) evaporated cane sugar (see Note on page 211)

5½ quarts (5.2 L) cold water

2 cups (470 ml) plain kombucha

1 kombucha SCOBY (page 216)

Find a location in your home that is away from direct sunlight and stays at a consistent temperature of 75º to 85ºF (24º to 29ºC), if possible. This is where you'll set up your 2½-gallon (9.5 L) porcelain vessel of kombucha to brew.

TO MAKE THE STARTER BATCH: Bring the 8 cups (1880 ml) water to a boil in a large-size pot, then add the loose tea equivalent. Allow the tea to steep for 5 minutes, then strain into a very large-size ceramic bowl. Add the sugar and stir until dissolved. Add the cold water and stir. The mixture should be room temperature at this point. Add the plain kombucha and stir again. Carefully pour the tea into the large-size porcelain vessel. Using clean hands, place the SCOBY on top of the tea. Cover with a tea towel and secure with a rubber band, in order to keep fruit flies out. Allow to sit for 1 week (away from other food that may attract fruit flies). Taste the tea. The ideal taste is only lightly sweet with a bit of tang but not overly vinegary. Keep tasting daily until the desired taste is achieved.

When the tea is to your liking, use the spigot to funnel half (1 gallon, or 3.8 L) into swing-top bottles or glass jars with

continued on next page

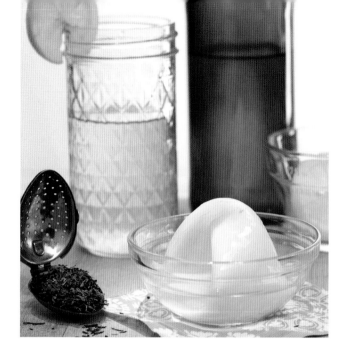

FOR REFILL BATCH:

4 cups (940 ml) water

4 tablespoons (32 g) loose black
  (or green) tea

1 cup (200 g) evaporated cane sugar

3 quarts (2.7 L) cold water

YIELD: 1 GALLON (3.8 L) PER WEEK

tight-fitting lids and refrigerate. Brew a refill batch as follows to replace bottled tea.

TO MAKE A REFILL BATCH: Bring the 4 cups (940 ml) water to a boil, then add the teabags or loose tea equivalent. Allow the tea to steep for 5 minutes, then strain into a large-size ceramic bowl. Add the sugar and stir until dissolved. Add the cold water, then pour into your existing vessel of kombucha, replenishing the tea that was bottled.

Allow the mixture to brew for 1 week before tasting. If not ready, continue to taste the tea daily until the desired taste is achieved. Continue to bottle and refill weekly, following the above instructions.

TO CLEAN THE VESSEL: Every 4 months, the vessel should be thoroughly cleaned. To do so, first remove the SCOBY and place it on a sheet tray. The SCOBY grows in layers during the 4 months of continuous brew. Discard, compost, or give away several of the bottom layers, which will be darker in color. A knife may be needed to separate the layers. You can also cut the SCOBY down to size if it has outgrown its jug. After trimming the SCOBY, place it in a bowl. Remove 2 cups (470 ml) of the kombucha and place in the bowl with the SCOBY.

Use the spigot to funnel and bottle all but the final 1 inch (2.5 cm) of liquid; this brownish, yeast-filled portion should be discarded in order to start fresh with a new population of yeast. (Because the spigot of most vessels is located at least 1 inch (2.5 cm) above the bottom of the vessel, it should not draw out the bottom settlement.)

Using a clean sponge and water, scrub the jug and spigot clean. Unscrew the spigot for a thorough cleaning. Scrub once more using distilled vinegar and rinse well.

With a clean vessel, a trimmed SCOBY, and 2 cups (470 ml) of reserved plain kombucha, restart the continuous brew process as outlined above.

RECIPE NOTES

• SCOBY is an acronym for symbiotic colony of bacteria and yeast.

• Be sure to consume the refrigerated kombucha within 1 month to prevent exploding bottles. If you'd like to keep it longer, simply store the kombucha in plastic containers instead.

• To create fizz in kombucha, add approximately 1 cup (235 ml) 100% fruit juice of choice to a clean, 2-liter plastic soda bottle. (The reason for plastic rather than glass is that in case of excess carbonation, the plastic will expand while the glass could crack.) Using a long wooden spoon, carefully peel the SCOBY away from one side of the jug and stir the kombucha to mix in the brownish yeast that lies at the bottom of the vessel; this yeast is the catalyst for the carbonation. Funnel brewed kombucha, plus any brown yeasty strands, into the 2-liter bottle, filling the bottle up to the tippy top. Screw on the cap tightly and set at room temperature for several days, until the plastic is taut and unyielding to the pressure of a squeeze, which indicates that gasses have built up in the bottle. At this point, refrigerate until consumption. And open carefully!

• Evaporated cane sugar, found in most grocery stores, carries a refinement that falls somewhere between white sugar, which is devoid of all minerals, and Sucanat (page 64), where the minerals are left untouched, leaving the rich brown color of the molasses intact. Evaporated cane sugar (or juice) contains only a very small amount of minerals and is light tan in color.

Living on a farm with 24 acres of lemons encourages one to acquire a killer lemonade recipe! By using a blender instead of heat to quickly emulsify the lemon and the honey, the beneficial enzymes and delicate nature of the unpasteurized raw honey are preserved. A very delicious, nutritious duo!

Apricot Lane Farms Lemonade >

1 cup (320 g) raw honey
1 cup (235 ml) freshly squeezed
   lemon juice
6 cups (1410 ml) water

In a blender, combine the honey and lemon juice. Blend on high for 30 seconds. Add the water and pulse to combine.

Refrigerate until chilled, then serve over ice.

YIELD: 8 CUPS (1880 ML)

There is something very satisfying about "building your own" anything. In the case of this recipe, I am thrilled knowing every ingredient in this milk is a word I can pronounce. In today's world of processed foods, that is just short of a miracle.

Creamy Almond Milk

3 cups (705 ml) water
1 cup (150 g) crunchy almonds
   (page 49)
1 teaspoon raw honey
½ teaspoon vanilla extract
Pinch sea salt

In the container of a high-speed blender, combine all the ingredients. Blend on high speed for 2 minutes. Strain through a chinois (page 83) and compost the pulp.

Rinse the blender and return the almond milk to it. Blend on high speed for 1 minute, then strain again through the chinois.

Almond milk can be served warm or chilled. Use within 4 days and be sure to shake well before pouring (separation is normal).

YIELD: 2¼ CUPS (530 ML)

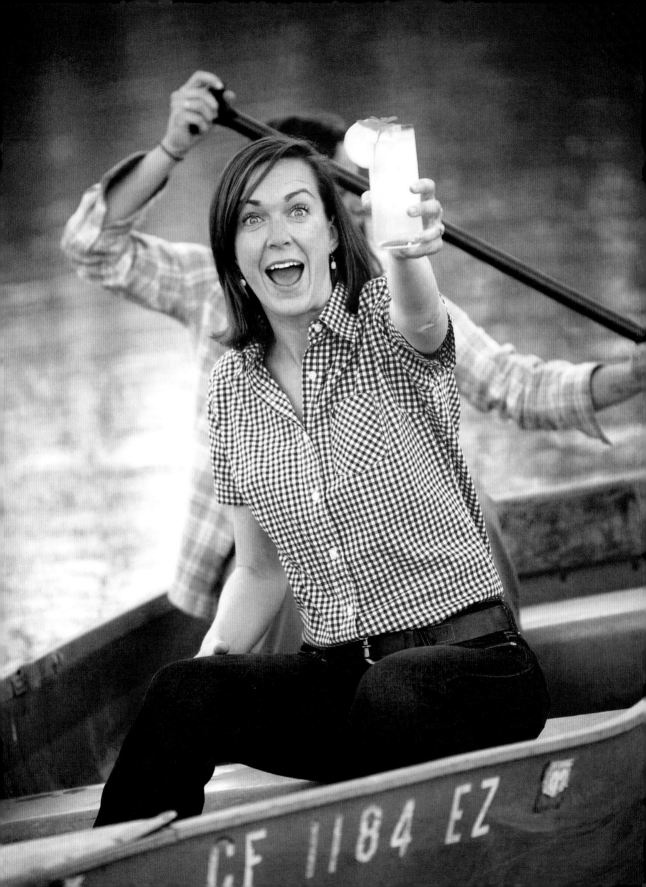

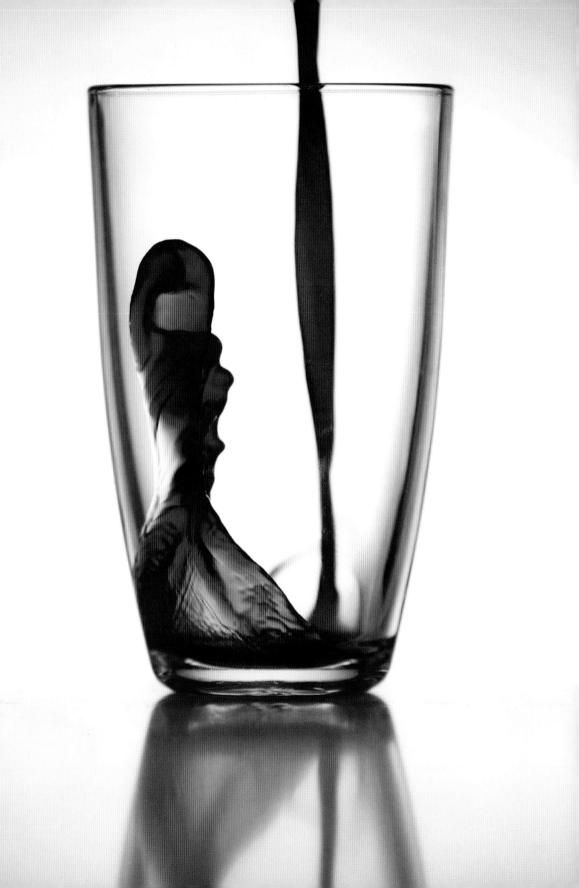

One 4-ounce (120 ml) glass of beet kvass morning and night serves as an excellent blood tonic, digestive regulator, blood alkalizer, liver cleanser, and overall healing tonic. In general, it keeps things moving! Remember, this is a detox tool, not a sugary beverage! The taste is acquired, and we find it most palatable when served cold. And if you're heading to a party tonight, avoid purple hands by wearing rubber gloves when peeling the beets!

Beet Kvass

Inspired by Sally Fallon

2 medium or 1 large beet

1 teaspoon sea salt

2 tablespoons (30 ml) whey (page 40)

YIELD: 2 QUARTS (1.8 L)

Peel the beets and chop into 1-inch (2.5 cm) chunks. Place in the bottom of a clean 1-quart (1 L) Mason jar. To the jar, add the sea salt and whey. Fill the jar with water up to 1 inch (2.5 cm) below the top. Put the lid on and shake thoroughly.

Leave the jar on the counter, at room temperature, for 2 days without opening, then transfer to the refrigerator to store. The jar does not need to be "burped."

Once chilled and ready to serve, carefully pour the desired amount into a glass, leaving the beets in the bottom of the jar to continue strengthening the liquid. Enjoy as a tonic beverage.

When all the liquid has been consumed, the process may be repeated one more time by adding the same amount of whey, sea salt, and water to the jar (which now only contains beets). Leave at room temperature for another 2 days without opening before transferring to the refrigerator for use.

When the second batch of liquid has been consumed, compost the beets and start fresh.

RECIPE NOTE

This recipe may easily be doubled. When doubling, use two 1-quart (940 ml) Mason jars (rather than one 2-quart [2 L] jar) in order to allow the jars to be rotated. When one jar is finished, begin the second round of fermentation with that jar while consuming the second jar. Kvass ripens beautifully over time. A couple of months of refrigerator time will produce an even richer and more probiotic-filled beverage—if you can wait that long!

RESOURCES

FATS AND OILS

BEEF TALLOW AND PORK LARD

U.S. Wellness Meats
www.grasslandbeef.com

BUTTER

Straus Family Creamery
http://strausfamilycreamery.com

COCONUT OIL

Tropical Traditions
www.tropicaltraditions.com

Wilderness Family Naturals
www.wildernessfamilynaturals.com

EXTRA-VIRGIN OLIVE OIL

Chaffin Family Orchards
www.chaffinfamilyorchards.com

GHEE

Pure Indian Foods
www.pureindianfoods.com

WALNUT OIL

La Nogalera
http://lanogalerawalnutoil.com

DAIRY AND EGGS

PASTURED EGGS

Find a farmer! Check out Local Harvest to find what's close.
www.localharvest.org

REAL MILK

Check out the Campaign for Real Milk and Real Milk Finder
www.realmilk.com

SUSTAINABLE MEAT, POULTRY, AND SEAFOOD

GRASS-FED BEEF

American Grassfed Association
www.americangrassfed.org

Novy Ranches
www.novyranches.com

PASTURED POULTRY

Tropical Traditions
www.tropicaltraditions.com

PORK, NITRATE-FREE BACON, HAM, AND MORE

U.S. Wellness Meats
www.grasslandbeef.com

SUSTAINABLE SEAFOOD

Marine Stewardship Council
www.msc.org

Seafood Watch, Monterey Bay Aquarium
www.montereybayaquarium.org/cr/seafoodwatch.aspx

Vital Choice (salmon roe)
www.vitalchoice.com

CULTURES

BUTTERMILK AND OTHER CULTURES

Cultures for Health
www.culturesforhealth.com

KEFIR GRAINS

Kefirlady
www.kefirlady.com

KOMBUCHA EQUIPMENT

Kombucha Kamp
www.kombuchakamp.com

POWDERED KEFIR STARTER

Body Ecology Diet
http://bodyecology.com

GRAIN

CORN

Anson Mills
http://ansonmills.com

Bread Beckers
www.breadbeckers.com

SPROUTED HARD RED AND HARD WHITE WHEAT BERRIES

To Your Health Sprouted Flour Company
www.organicsproutedflour.net

UNSPROUTED HARD RED, HARD WHITE, AND SOFT WHITE WHEAT BERRIES

Bread Beckers
www.breadbeckers.com

SWEETENERS

COCONUT SUGAR

Wilderness Family Naturals
www.wildernessfamilynaturals.com

MAPLE SYRUP

Find it locally if you can. Check out
Local Harvest to find what's close.
www.localharvest.org

Trader Joe's brand Organic
Maple Syrup
www.traderjoes.com

MAPLE SYRUP AND
MAPLE SUGAR

Coombs Family Farms
www.coombsfamilyfarms.com

POWDERED GREEN STEVIA

Frontier
www.frontiercoop.com

RAW HONEY

Really Raw Honey
www.reallyrawhoney.com

Honey Pacifica
www.honeypacifica.com

SUCANAT, HONEY GRAN-
ULES, AND POWDERED
HONEY GRANULES

Bread Beckers
www.breadbeckers.com

OTHER

TOMATO PRODUCTS

Muir Glen, BPA-free cans
www.muirglen.com

Eden Organics, Crushed tomatoes
in glass jars
www.edenfoods.com

COCONUT AMINOS

Coconut Secret
www.coconutsecret.com

FERMENTED GREEN
CABBAGE SAUERKRAUT

Farmhouse Culture
http://farmhouseculture.com

Goldmine Natural Food Co.
www.goldminenaturalfoods.com

FISH SAUCE

Red Boat
www.redboatfishsauce.com

GRASS-FED GELATIN

Bernard Jensen International
www.bernardjensen.com

Great Lakes Gelatin
www.greatlakesgelatin.com

KOMBU

Eden Organic
www.edenfoods.com

LOOSE-LEAF TEA

Mountain Rose Herbs
www.mountainroseherbs.com

MAYONNAISE

Wilderness Family Naturals
www.wildernessfamilynaturals.com

PICKLING LIME

Mrs. Wages
www.mrswages.com

SHOPPING GUIDE

Weston A. Price Foundation
Shopping Guide
www.westonaprice.org/about-
the-foundation/shopping-guide

SOY-FREE CHICKEN/
POULTRY FEED

Magill Ranch & Cascade Feeds
www.magillranch.com

Modesto Milling
www.modestomilling.com

EQUIPMENT

DEHYDRATORS

Excalibur
www.excaliburdehydrator.com

GRAIN MILLS

Bread Beckers
www.breadbeckers.com

Komo Grain Mills
www.grainmillshop.com

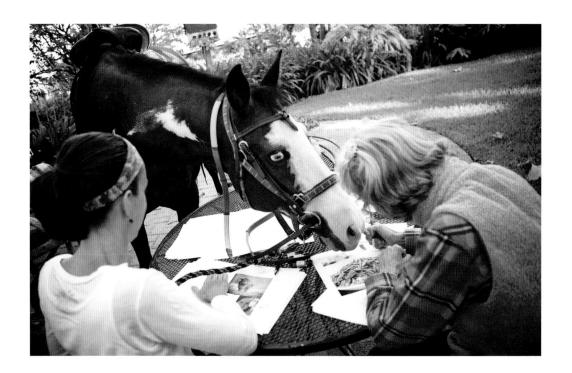

OUR THANKS!

In the fall of 2009, this cookbook idea was born. Countless generous people supported our creative process and weathered the never-ending feeling that comes with finishing a book.

Specific thanks to Damon Morda; Matt and Megan Schrecengost; Paul and Jessica Gurinas; Beck Hansen; Sally Fallon; the team at Fair Winds Press, especially Amanda Waddell and Winnie Prentiss; Anna Robertson; Betty Merti; Jayne Ward; and Ian Berry; the *Back to Butter* photography team; and the hardworking staff at Apricot Lane Farms.

And finally, thank you to the two who ate the most butter of all—Dave Schrecengost and John Chester.

ABOUT THE AUTHORS

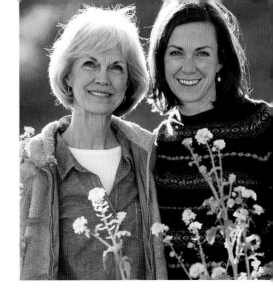

Molly Chester began her career in the entertainment industry, as an on-air producer for the primetime A&E original series, *Random 1*. Soon after, she moved to the Big Apple to attend The Natural Gourmet Institute of Health & Culinary Arts. Following an internship at Gramercy Park's raw food restaurant, Pure Food & Wine, she began private cheffing, prompting a move to Los Angeles with her husband, documentary filmmaker and photographer, John Chester. Molly immediately secured several high-profile clients, and her cheffing and teaching services became recommended by progressive doctors and dentists, who prescribed Traditional Foods techniques to heal their patients.

Molly has spoken at Harvard Business School on *How to Unleash the Healing Power of Food*. Most recently, she and John began farming a 160-acre (6.4 ha) beautiful plot of land in Moorpark, CA. Apricot Lane Farms is a stunning organic and biodynamic farming project that includes pastured chickens, cows, sheep, ducks, and over seventy-five varieties of fruit trees. It is being designed to provide a voice and a platform to traditional and ecological farming techniques, while experimenting to make these techniques commercially viable. John Chester's short films about Apricot Lane Farms are now regularly featured on the talk show *Super Soul Sunday* on Oprah Winfrey Network's, OWN.

Oh, and perhaps most importantly, Molly grew up sitting on the kitchen counter of this next lovely lady ...

As a young girl, in rural Pennsylvania, **Sandy Schrecengost** helped her ailing mother by climbing a wooden stool to prepare simple family meals. That experience, coupled with a beloved grandmother who understood garden-to-table cooking, planted a passion in Sandy to one day nurture her own family wirh food. Before marrying and becoming a mother of two, she spent years as a public school teacher, coaching dance and gymnastics.

Then, in the mid '70s, Sandy stepped out of the schoolhouse and into the kitchen, devoting the next thirty years to putting nurturing meals on the family dinner table. To her dismay, she gradually discovered convenient, processed ingredients of her generation may have been nurturing, but not *nourishing*. In an effort to reverse the decline of her family's health, Sandy took a fresh look at her pantry and began championing traditional foods and their proper preparation as key to restoration and maintenance of health.

Sandy currenlty lives in Atlanta with her husband, David, and remains committed to using her gift of teaching to share her story about the power of traditional foods. She enjoys translating that love of Traditional Foods into sound bites that appeal and apply to real families. Sandy is convinced a dash of common sense and a collection of real food recipes can be catalysts for change. *Back to Butter* is her offering toward that transformation.

For more information, visit Apricot Lane Farms at http://www.apricotlanefarms.com/ and Molly and Sandy's blog at http://www.organicspark.com/.

INDEX